ACCEPTANCE AND COMMITMENT THERAPY

THE ULTIMATE GUIDE TO BREAK FREE FROM FEARS, ANXIETY AND WORRY

James Parker

The information provided herein is stated to be truthful and consistent, in that any liability, in terms of inattention or otherwise, by any usage or abuse of any policies, processes, or directions contained within is the solitary and utter responsibility of the recipient reader. Under no

circumstances will any legal responsibility or blame be held against the publisher for any reparation, damages, or monetary loss due to the information herein, either directly or indirectly.

Respective authors own all copyrights not held by the publisher.

The information herein is offered for informational purposes solely, and is universal as so. The presentation of the information is without contract or any type of guarantee assurance. The trademarks that are used are without any consent, and the publication of the trademark is without permission or backing by the trademark owner. All trademarks and brands within this book are for clarifying purposes only and are the owned by the owners themselves, not affiliated with this document.

DISCLAIMER

The information in this eBook, whether provided in audio version hardcopy or digitally is for general information purposes and nothing contained in it is, or is intended to be construed as advice. It is not a substitute for medical attention, treatment, examination, advice, treatment of existing conditions or diagnosis and is not intended to provide a clinical diagnosis nor take the place of proper medical advice from a fully qualified medical practitioner. You are responsible for consulting a suitable medical professional before using any of the eBook's information , before trying any treatment or taking any course of action that may directly or indirectly affect your health or well-being.

CHAPTER 1

WHAT IS ACT?

Acceptance and commitment therapy (ACT) trains uprightness aptitudes to assist individuals with living and carry on in a manner that is reliable with individual qualities while creating mental adaptability. ACT expert's assist people with perceiving ways they make difficulties in their endeavors to stifle, oversee, and control enthusiastic encounters.

Through identifying these obstacles and solving them, people can become better able to make space for values-based acts that promote wellness.

HISTORY OF ACT

For decades, psychology researchers have been working to develop time-limited, science-based interventions for people who want to overcome mental health conditions. As a result, many people have had substantial success in addressing and managing a range of concerns and, as a result, experiencing greater well-being. By the by, long haul recuperation and counteraction of backslide are as yet huge as zones of potential trouble for those looking for psychological well-being treatments.New kinds of treatments have as of late been created, including ACT, with expectations of expanding long haul accomplishment in treating emotional wellness conditions.

ACT depends on social system hypothesis (RFT), an examination school concentrated on human language and discernment. RFT demonstrates the human brain's thinking capacities in taking care of issues that might be ineffective in helping individuals settle mental agony. Based on this recommendation, ACT treatment was created with the point of instructing individuals that albeit mental agony is ordinary, by moving the manner in which we consider torment, we can learn approaches to live more beneficial, more full lives.

Starting in the late 1990s, many nitty-gritty consideration guides were made to detail techniques for utilizing ACT to treat diverse emotional wellness conditions. Treatment using these manuals was tentatively inspected and reinforced the use of ACT in treating substance abuse, psychosis, strain, distress, unending anguish, and dietary issues.

UNDERSTANDING THE THEORY OF ACT

ACT hypothesis doesn't characterize the manifestations or issues of undesirable passionate encounters. Or maybe, it attempts to deliver a few people's propensities to see people looking for treatment as harmed or imperfect, and plans to assist individuals with understanding life's completion and essentialness. That completion incorporates a wide range of human life, including the subsequent enduring that follows certain conditions.

ACT does not attempt to change or discourage negative thoughts or feelings explicitly (as is the case for cognitive behavioral therapy) but rather helps people to develop a fresh and caring interaction with these interactions. The move will free people from challenges trying to control their interactions and make them become more responsive to behaviors that are compatible with their beliefs, the interpretation of values, and the identification of values-based goals that are also key components of ACT.

SIX CORE PROCESSES OF ACT

Psychological flexibility, ACT's main aim, usually occurs through several core processes.

Developing imaginative hopelessness means discussing previous attempts to solve or avoid the problems that would lead an adult to seek counseling. Through acknowledging the workability or lack of workability of these efforts, ACT creates opportunities for people to act in a way that is more compatible with what matters most to them.

Acknowledgment of one's enthusiastic experience can be portrayed as the way toward figuring out how to encounter the scope of human feelings with a point of view that is thoughtful, open, and adequate.The way toward characterizing what is generally significant throughout everyday life and of explaining how one wishes to live is to pick esteemed life bearings.Taking action may apply to one's commitment to making improvements and participating in actions that drive one toward what is most respected.

Such systems are intertwined and interacting and not distinct. All these mechanisms are implemented and established by direct experiences that the individual in counseling recognizes and engages in over the duration of the procedure. Psychological flexibility can simply be defined as' the ability to be present, to open up, and to do what matters.'

MINDFULNESS AND ACT

Mindfulness can be described as keeping in touch with the present moment rather than drifting off into automatic piloting. Mindfulness allows an individual to communicate with the self-observing, the portion which is conscious but different from the self-observation. Care techniques additionally assist people with expanding consciousness of every one of the five detects, just as their contemplations and feelings.ACT does not attempt to change or discourage negative thoughts or feelings explicitly but rather helps people to develop a fresh and respectful engagement with those interactions.

Also, mindfulness increases the ability of an individual to detach themselves from thoughts. Challenges relating to painful feelings, urges, or situations are often reduced first and eventually accepted afterward. Acceptance is the desire to encourage internal and external interaction to take place, rather than resisting or preventing the encounter. If someone says, "I'm a terrible person," the person may be asked to say then, "I'm feeling I'm a terrible person." It actually removes the subject from the thought, thereby removing them of their negative charge.

When people experience painful emotions, such as anxiety, they may be instructed to open up, breathe in, or make room for anxiety's physical feeling and allow it to stay there as it is, without exacerbating or minimizing it.

VALUES CLARIFICATION AND ACT

The explanation of qualities can help individuals characterize what is generally significant—their qualities, as it were—and make a compelling move that is guided by those qualities. For expansion, psychological well-being proficiency may utilize various exercises to help distinguish wanted standards for those in treatment. Regularly these standards fill in as a guide in the way of intentional and effective activities.Investigating excruciating feelings or overthinking an issue can meddle with one's capacity to pick intentional, esteem driven activity.Through deliberately freeing individuals from this task, ACT will encourage people to act more in accordance with their beliefs and live in a way that feels natural and satisfying.

WHO ARE THOS THAT PLAY ACT OFFERS?

To clinicians who want to provide this type of therapy, the ACT group does not provide official certification. The Contextual Behavior Science Society (ACBS) operates a national list of participants who have listed themselves as ACT practitioners, and this register may be a good place for those interested in finding an ACT practitioner to continue.

The ACBS likewise gives recommendations to those keen on finding an ACT specialist: Contact the branch of brain research, social work, or psychiatry at a close-by school or college. Employees or laborers who are masters in conduct treatment or intellectual social treatment might be familiar with a close-by ACT pro.

The Association for Behavioral and Cognitive Therapy's United States-based site keeps up a rundown of the conduct and intellectual treatment suppliers. These advisors may likewise give ACT or may know about an associate giving ACT.

In nations other than the United States, ABCT-like associations might be a decent spot to search for suppliers that convey ACT or that can allude advisors prepared in ACT.

SIX ACCEPTANCE AND COMMITMENT THERAPY PRINCIPLES

The following are six essential standards type of Acceptance and Commitment Therapies. They cooperate towards the primary objectives of taking care of agonizing contemplations and encounters successfully and making a rich, crucial life.

The ideas are:
- Expansion and acceptance
- Contact and connection with the present moment

- The Observing Self
- Values clarification
- Committed action (Harris, 2006; Harris, 2007)

LETS first take a brief glance at what they mean.

Standard 1: Cognitive defusion

This ability is tied in with figuring out how to see musings, pictures, recollections and different comprehensions for what they are–just bits of language and pictures than what they frequently seem, by all accounts, to be: undermining occasions, decisions that must be complied, or target certainties and realities.

The inverse mental procedure intellectual combination alludes to a blend of perceptions (mental items, for example, considerations, pictures, or recollections) with the things they allude to. For instance, in intellectual combination, our brain could have a similar response to the expression "chocolate cake" as though we were given a cut of it. That is, the basic appearance of the boosts the words "chocolate cake"– may serve to begin us slobbering, envisioning the sweet taste, and feeling the thick, smooth surface in our icing hands. In a psychological combination state, it appears as though:

Musings are reality: as though what we believe is really occurring.

Considerations are reality: we thoroughly trust them.

Considerations are significant: we treat them genuinely, we give them our complete consideration.

Insights are orders: we subsequently obey them.

Examinations are wise: we acknowledge that they know best, and we follow their suggestion.

Examinations are perils: We let them alert us or upset us (Harris, 2007) But, as any well-being nourishment nut can tell you, the word or image of a chocolate cake isn't comparable to the real thing (at any rate similar to both pleasure and caloric affirmation!).

The subjective defusion process is planned for isolating terrible, unwelcome contemplations, sentiments, urges, recollections, or other mental items from ourselves. It is the progression over from them (a procedure called disidentification in customs like Psychosynthesis-Assagioli, 1973/1984) to get a view and perceive the truth about them: only a smidgen.

Standard 2: Expansion/acknowledgment

This is otherwise called "acknowledgment" by some other ACT clinicians and researchers, Harris term this capacity "development" on the grounds that different definitions are loaded up with "acknowledgment." This alludes to the act of preparing for upsetting emotions, discernments, and motivations, instead of endeavoring to stifle or drive them away. We notice that they irritate us significantly less by opening up and permitting them to travel every which way without managing them, fleeing from them, or offering them pointless treatment. They likewise move quicker, as opposed to simply sticking around and irritating us (Harris, 2006; Harris, 2007).

Envision the circumstance for the shopper who states, "I am so apprehensive to go out on the town. I'm reluctant to such an extent that I must state anything, or that I'm going to state something extremely moronic. "By using CBT techniques, we as advisors could help the client dispute the negative beliefs that she's a poor conversationalist or a boring date, replacing her anxious thoughts with positive ones, affirming ones like that she's interesting, good at conversation, or a worthy social partner. Through longer, psychotherapeutic cycles, we have been able to help her uncover the events in her history (probably early childhood) that produced her sense of social ineptitude. However, psychotherapy takes a long time, and even when the effect of past history on present experience becomes known, there is still the "war of words" as the different voices-the critical ones and the affirming ones-call for attention. Being in a war like that is a huge drain of resources!

The expansion/acceptance principle of ACT works differently. It would expect the customer to think she'll be going out on a date. She would then be told to check her body, determining where she most felt the fear. Let's say she's reporting she is experiencing a huge lump in her throat. She may then be approached to watch the irregularity's sensation as though she were a researcher who had never observed anything like it: seeing its shape, weight, vibration, temperature, throb, and different viewpoints.She would be invited to breathe into the lump, make room for it, allowing it to be there (although we'd be highly empathetic in understanding she didn't like it or wanted it there!). She may be offered the "homework" in treatments to practice monitoring the lump of anxiety: not trying to get rid of it but just having the lump sense, and probably other anxiety-related stimuli, come and go as they please: accept them, not fight them, but also not pursue them.

Principle 3: Contact (association) with the present minute

To permit ourselves to encounter the sensations, emotions, and contemplations that have emerged is to follow the third ACT standard, that of reaching the present minute, which Harris likes to call "association" (Harris, 2007, p 47). This involves living in the present, reflecting on whatever we do, and taking full awareness of the reality of here and now: with transparency, curiosity, and receptivity. As opposed to choosing not to move on or agonizing over what's to come, we're profoundly associated with what's happening directly here in the present moment. We're completely occupied with whatever we do with association.

We could ask in practicing connection: why bother to pull ourselves out of the past or the future to return to the present moment? Why is that deemed so beneficial to us? Harris points to three main reasons: This is the main life we have (in any event, for some, who have confidence in ideas, for example, rebirth, this is the main life we know about or will, in general, have data about the present moment), so why not benefit as much as possible from that? Being just half-present is missing a large portion of that. Lack of current-moment interaction is analogous to listening to a beloved piece of music with earplugs in the ears, or enjoying a favorite food when the mouth is still sore from a dentist's visit; we lack the richness that might be there.

Considering that an ACT structure is dedicated to effective, value-driven intervention, we should inform clients that, in order to create a meaningful life, we need to take action, and the power to act only resides at this time. As the Arab saying goes, "It is difficult to lift a camel that has not yet reached (the future), nor one that has departed (the past)."

"Action" means effective action and not just any old action. Effective action is defined in ACT as the one that helps us move in a valued direction. In order to find out how that direction lies, we have to be psychologically present to be aware of what's going on, how we're reacting, and, therefore, how we're right to respond. Harris recommends recalling a mnemonic for ACT: "Consider and be present in your inner experience; choose a respected direction; and take action."

Indeed, even the individuals who will, in general, live their lives through the intervening impact of their considerations, for the most, part have some present-minute contact understanding: times when it emerges precipitously and surprisingly.For starters, the client anticipating social ineptitude could be prompted to focus on any moment she might have been totally absorbed in being with someone else (date or otherwise): the memory of, say, holding on every word the individual said, noting the gestures their mouth produced as they spoke, recognizing the person's smell, and how their hair was (or not) peeled. Full engagement with another person is likely to have ejected thoughts of social inadequacy from her mind (though temporarily).

It isn't important to go on a genuine date to rehearse this expertise (on account of the individual who fears social uncouthness), or even have someone else around. Be that as it may, we can establish ourselves right now, just by tuning in. For example, an ACT counsel may demand that a client notice every little piece of their experience of tidying up: the assessment of the water as it hits the skin and runs down, seeing the rising steam in the washroom, or the smell of any chemicals or various things that are applied to the body during the showering or after-shower care process. Or then again an individual could practice the present-minute affiliation standard by watching minute nuances of the after-dinner dishwashing experience: the ringing sound of the plates against the seat top, the feeling of the sudsy water washing over them, the sensation and sound of squeaking as the things become truly great, and the visual experience of putting them on the channel.Even easier: an ACT-oriented advisor could give a customer a single piece of food–say, a dried fig–and ask the person to concentrate on nothing but eating it. The client may be encouraged to establish intrusive thoughts and feelings; these may be allowed to come and go as they will; the concentration of the client will remain focused on the fruit. After "graduating" to a relational circumstance, a customer, for example, we were talking about would be urged to have a discussion with someone else concentrating completely on that individual as opposed to on their own contemplations and notions. Anyway the association/contact occurs with the present minute, it occurs through the Observing Self.

Principle 4: Observing Self
The Observing Self is an important aspect of human consciousness, which Modern philosophy largely

ignores. To associate with it is to approach an extraordinary feeling of self: a progression of cognizance that is perpetual, ever-present, and unequipped for hurt.From this most holistic view of oneself, it is possible to experience explicitly these claims as contained in some relaxations in body-feelings-ment that, "I am my flesh, and I am more than my body; I am my emotions, and I am more than my feelings; I am my spirit, but then I am more than my brain" (Palmer, 1997). From this position, we will understand that our emotions, perceptions, experiences, desires, sensations, pictures, positions, and physical body are secondary facets of ourselves, but they are not the core of who we are, because they are constantly changing.

To understand the Observing Self principle is to understand that, when we become conscious of our thoughts, two processes actually occur: that of thinking and that of observing the thinking. We can draw the consideration of the customer to the qualification between the musings that emerge and the self that watches them-over and over if essential.No inner experience (that is: thought, feeling, image, or urge) is dangerous or controlling from the Observing Self perspective.

We have stated earlier that the six principles work together to help us build a meaningful life. We can now state that the present-moment-connection with the Observing Self happens. This involves bringing our complete attention to what's going on here and now, without becoming overwhelmed or affected by the self of thought. Through definition, the Observing Self is said to be non-judgmental, since decisions are emotions, and thus a result of the self-thinking. The Observing Self is not wrestling with reality; it sees things as they are without resisting it. It is only by judging things like "bad," "unfair," or "mean" that we resist them. At that point, it's simply the reasoning that discloses to us that "life shouldn't resemble it (the truth) is," that in the event that we were elsewhere, elsewhere, or by one way or another extraordinary, we would be more joyful. It is consequently our self we've envisioned that creates dreams ourselves and life, withdrawing us from reality through exhaustion, interference, or obstacle.

Alternately, the Observing Self is unequipped for obstruction or fatigue.It welcomes every stimulus, every experience with open-mindedness, curiosity, and interest. Boredom and resistance are cycles of thought: tales that would make life more interesting or easier "if."The Observing Self, ever-present and accessible, can slice through that, awakening us and associating us to the unending prospects of human experience we may experience, regardless of whether the experience is new or natural.Paradoxically, by engaging the Observing Self as we encounter unpleasant experiences, we often find the aspects we were afraid of becoming far less troubling than they had been before. They see things in a new way.

Interfacing with the Observing Self methods means having the prepared ability to perceive from agony and misery.As we remain in the shoes of the (disidentified) Observing Self, we can, in any case, feel agony and despondency (our reasoning self may even now give us considerations that we hurt or are despondent), however not the entirety of our awareness is bound in that, since some of it includes the Observing Self in watching us feel the torment. Along these lines, the experience turns out to be progressively endurable as we experience an increasingly open mind, by picking two situations in which to be.

Inside the setting of some random experience, we can pick where we stand—either intentionally or unknowingly, naturally. Our decision is controlled by the qualities that we hold, so being clear about what those qualities are is a key part of compelling living.

Rule 5: Values explanation

This ACT rule is tied in with explaining what the most significant thing we can access in the most profound piece of ourselves is.It involves asking what kind of person we want to be, what makes sense to us, and what we want to stand for in this lifetime. Our values guide our lives and motivate us to make significant changes. Guided by values, not only do we experience a greater sense of purpose and joy, but we also see that even when "bad" things happen to us, life can be rich and meaningful!

ACT-oriented therapy could, therefore, encourage the participant to complete a questionnaire on "life values," which requires respondents to focus on their principles in ten fields, from family and marriage relationships to group life and relationship with nature through schooling and spirituality. Many consumers may like to miss clarity tasks around principles, and there may be many explanations why this is so.

Values vs. targets
Many individuals might not be clear on the difference between principles and goals. Harris argues why ambitions are a one-shot deal when ideals are so, because they are everything we hold dear constantly in our lives. He uses someone's analogy that goes on a journey, saying he's going to keep going west. That steady heading is practically equivalent to a worth, in light of the fact that regardless of how far the individual goes, there is constantly an all the more westerly bearing wherein he can continue.Saying he intends to climb to the peak of a particular mountain along the way, however, is a goal, because once he climbs to the top of the mountain, he has reached the goal, and it's a done deal. When we realize what we want, we're able to derive concrete expectations and

live through our beliefs. But another clean obstacle to enacting this principle may lie therein.

Principle 5

But are they true values to me? A number of persons may resist enacting or even completing any questionnaires around it because they are uncertain whether their "real" values will reflect the answers they provide. Of course, just because somebody thinks they respect a particular thing –say, being loving–it can be regarded as their interest because, by nature, a value is something that we love. The response to why we value something above all is simply to respect it, to have it as an interest. This is an assertion close to the person who says... I don't know what I want. Once, whatever we choose is our interest, merely because we've recognized it by name. But it does raise the question of... What if my values conflict? If you're probably working to help clients use ACT methodologies, you'll consider this one; it's true. It is hard to unimaginable not to have values pulling one in various ways, particularly in wild present-day life. For example, a client can past a sensible uncertainty regard the essentialness of significant worth time with family, and correspondingly as significantly need to rise through the positions occupied with working, concentrating on that; at some stage, if not routinely, the two characteristics are most likely going to battle.

Actually, once in a while, we need to organize one space over another, asking ourselves: "What is generally significant in my life as of now, given the clashing qualities that I experience?" The individual should then follow up on the picked esteem, without stressing over what the person in question passes up, realizing that at some later stage, if important, the parity can be" amended. In any case, some will protest their qualities being explained based on past disappointment or dissatisfaction.

I would incline toward not to talk about it; I'm just setting myself up for guile. The individuals who have encountered a lot of disappointment or inability to live picked qualities might be reluctant to recognize what they truly need, for dread that they will neglect to accomplish it–once more. Such twin challenges to the option of simple principles refer to the "I can't alter," "I'll always lose," or "I don't deserve any better" doubts that exist in many minds. The past is the past, and it can not be altered, but the future is just now starting. Clients voicing this kind of reluctance may be advised to relax in their frustration and accept that these comments are pure thoughts; they will come and go as the client refocuses on the useful workout.

I am going to do that later. Yeah... Okay. You'll certainly have heard this one before as a counselor or other mental health helper! Principle 5 on the clarification of values will go nowhere when the beast of procrastination roams. Explain to the person that it's now "later," so time to do what's enshrined in the very name of ACT therapy.

Principle 6:

Committed behavior
The person sets targets and acts upon this last principle: but not just any action. Here the individual comprehends that the rich and significant life he/she needs is made through a powerful activity, which is guided by the qualities picked.Will the followers have a perfect record of pursuing the objectives they set? No, of course not, but the values are there to provide inspiration and motivation for re-engaging action, no matter how many times someone may go "off the rails"–or not even get down the track. The targets are there to inform the person of the acts that will help him or her achieve the visualized existence. In the end, it's up to each person to provide the will and energy to take action.

In the would-be traveler who really, really needs to go to Asia, we will consider comparison. The person buys books about Africa for details and tour guides, hires travel agents, and prepares the itinerary for the specific spots he wants to visit. He is sure that his life will be awesome in the event that he can simply find a workable pace! In any case, truth be told, he won't be available toward the day's end for any of his arranged safaris–and nothing will change in his life–except if he escapes the rocker, gathers his sack, and faces up on the named day to take the plane in. No measure of finding out about Africa will give him the real African experience he wants. At last, he should supply the will and vitality to go there to be changed by Africa's rich and significant experience.

CHAPTER 2

THE CLEAR EXPALNATION ON ACCEPTANCE AND COMMITMENT THERAPY (ACT), COGNITIVE-BEHAVIORAL (CBT), ARE THEY EVIDENCE-BASED?

Envision a treatment that doesn't endeavor to lessen side effects in any case, as a side-effect, gets indication decrease.A therapy firmly rooted in the tradition of empirical science, yet with great emphasis on values, forgiveness, acceptance, compassion, living in the present moment, and having access to a transcendent sense of oneself. A treatment so difficult to define that it has been defined as an "existential humanistic cognitive behavioral therapy." Acceptance and commitment therapy, known as "ACT" (pronounced as the term "act"), is a behavioral therapy focused on an awareness that contradicts most Traditional psychology's ground rules. It utilizes a diverse blend of abilities in analogy, Catch 22, and care, alongside a wide exhibit of experiential activities and qualities, drove conduct mediations.ACT has been shown to be successful with a number of psychiatric conditions: insomnia, ADHD, occupational tension, chronic pain, terminal cancer trauma, anxiety, PTSD, anorexia, opioid addiction, drug misuse, and even schizophrenia.[1] A report by Bach & Hayes[2] found that with only four hours of ACT, hospital re-entry levels among schizophrenic patients fell by 50 percent over the next six months.

ACT'S GOAL

ACT's goal is to create a vibrant and meaningful life, while at the same time acknowledging the suffering that ultimately follows it. "ACT" is a good abbreviation, because this therapy is about taking effective action that is guided by our deepest values and in which we are fully involved. We can only build a meaningful life by conscientious practice. Of course, when we try to create such an existence, we can face all sorts of obstacles, in the form of uncomfortable and unwelcome "private encounters" (thought, picture, emotion, feeling, desire, and memory). ACT acquires awareness skills as an effective way of dealing with those private experiences.

WHAT IS MINDFULNESS?

At the point when I converse with customers about care, I characterize it as: "Deliberately carrying attention to your experience at this very moment with transparency, intrigue, and receptivity. There are numerous aspects to care: remembering living for the present minute; connecting completely in what you do, as opposed to "getting lost" in your considerations; and permitting your emotions to be as they seem to be, allowing them to travel every which way, as opposed to attempting to control them. Indeed, even the most horrible feelings, observations, improvements, and pictures can appear to be less upsetting or overpowering when we see our private experiences with trustworthiness and responsiveness. Mindfulness would thus be able to assist us with changing our collaboration with awful contemplations and emotions in a manner that decreases their effect and impact on our lives.

HOW DOES ACT VARY FROM OTHER APPROACHES FOCUSED ON MINDFULNESS?

ACT is one of the supposed "third waves" of social treatments—alongside Dialectical Behavior Therapy (DBT), Mindfulness-Based Cognitive Therapy (MBCT), and Mindfulness-Based Stress Reduction (MBSR)—all of which place extraordinary accentuation on the advancement of care abilities.

Introduced by Steve Hayes in 1986, ACT was the first of such "third wave" interventions and now has a comprehensive collection of scientific data to support its efficacy. In the fifties and sixties, the "first phase" of therapeutic therapy concentrated on explicit behavioral change and used strategies related to operational and traditional conditioning concepts.

In many respects, ACT differs from DBT, MBCT, and MBSR. For example, MBSR and MBCT are basically manualized therapy procedures, intended for use with stress and depression care units. DBT is usually a mixture of social skills training and individual therapy, specifically designed to treat Borderline Personality Disorder in a population. Interestingly, ACT can be utilized in a wide scope of clinical populaces with people, couples, and gatherings, both as a brief treatment or as long haul treatment. In fact, instead of adopting a manualized procedure, ACT encourages the practitioner to build and individualize their own mindfulness techniques, or even co-create them for clients. ACT is the only Modern psychotherapy produced in accordance with its own basic human language and perception study project.

Another major difference is that ACT sees formal awareness meditation as only one of many ways to teach awareness skills. Mindfulness abilities are "divided" into four sub-sets:
- Acceptance
- Cognitive defusion
- Communication with the present moment
- The Observing Self
- The spectrum of ACT approaches to improve these skills is broad and continues to grow, spanning from conventional breath mediation to cognitive defusion.

WHAT'S UNIQUE IN ACT?

ACT is the only Western psychotherapy founded in tandem with its own basic human language and perception research program-Relational Framework

Theory (RFT). Nonetheless, looking through RFT in depth is beyond the reach of this paper.

As a conspicuous difference to most Western psychotherapy, ACT has no decrease in manifestations as an objective. ACT has no decrease in manifestations as an objective. This depends on the view that the progressing endeavor to free "manifestations" in any case really makes a clinical issue. When a private encounter is marked as a "manifestation," a battle is made with the "side effect." An "indication" is something "obsessive" by definition, and something we ought to be attempting to dispose of. In ACT, the point is to change our relationship with our troublesome contemplations and sentiments, so we never again see them as "side effects." Instead, we figure out how to see them as innocuous mental occasions, regardless of whether they are awkward and transient. Amusingly, it is through this procedure that ACT really accomplishes a decrease in side effects—yet as a result and not as an objective.

Positive Normality

One perspective in which ACT is uncommon is that it doesn't depend on the reason of "positive typicality." The modern way of thinking depends on the presumption of stable ordinariness: that by definition, people are mentally sound, and with a solid situation, way of life, and social setting (with "self-realization" openings), people ought to just be agreeable and mollified. Mental experiencing this point of view is viewed as strange, an infection or disorder driven by unordinary neurotic procedures.

How can it be that ACT presumes this supposition that isn't right? On the off chance that we take a gander at the measurements, we find that just about 30 % or the grown-up populace will experience the ill effects of a perceived mental issue in any year. The World Health Organization estimates that depression is currently the fourth-largest, most expensive and most debilitating disease in the world, and will be the second-largest by 2020. One-tenth of the grown-up populace experiences clinical discouragement at whatever week, and one out of five individuals will experience the ill effects of it sooner or later in their lifetime. What's more, one of every four grown-ups will experience the ill effects of medication or liquor fixation at some phase of their lifetime. There are presently in excess of twenty million heavy drinkers in the U.S. alone.5 More alarming and calming is the finding that almost one of every two individuals will experience a phase of life when they genuinely consider suicide and will battle with it for about fourteen days or more. Nonetheless, perceive the numerous kinds of mental enduring that don't speak to "wellbeing conditions"— discouragement, separation, estrangement, uselessness, low confidence, social dread, and agony related with so many points as dogmatism, segregation, sexism, abusive behavior at home, and separation. Obviously, in spite of the fact that our way of life in written history is higher than at any other time, there is mental enduring surrounding us.

Dangerous Normality

ACT accepts that a typical human brain's mental procedures are regularly damaging and eventually make mental languishing over us all. Besides, ACT hypothesizes that the wellspring of this wretchedness is simply the jargon of man. Human language is an exceptionally mind-boggling image framework, with words, pictures, sounds, outward appearances, and physical motions in it. They utilize that jargon in two areas: private and open. Open language use includes perusing, talking, imitating, signaling, drawing, painting, performing, moving, and so on. Private language utilization incorporates thinking, envisioning, staring off into space, arranging, picturing, and so forth. An increasingly specialized term for the private utilization of language is "comprehension." Now obviously, the brain isn't a "thing" or an "object." Rather, it is a mind-boggling set of subjective procedures, for example, examination, correlation, assessment, arranging, recollecting, representation — and these procedures depend on human language.Thus in ACT, the term "conscious" is used as a symbol for human language itself. ACT implies that a normal human mind's psychological processes are often harmful and sooner or later cause psychological suffering for all of us.

The most amazing part is that human language is a double edged sword. On the constructive, it encourages us to make world maps and models; to foresee and get ready for the future; to share information; to gain from an earlier time; to envision things that have never existed and to keep making them; to create decides that adequately direct our conduct and help us flourish as a network; to speak with individuals who are far away; and to gain from individuals who never again live.

The clouded side of language is that we use it to lie, control, and misdirect; to spread defamation, criticism, and obliviousness; to impel despise, partiality, and savagery; to make weapons of mass demolition, and mass contamination enterprises; to harp on and "remember" past agonizing occasions; to be reluctant to envision terrible fates; to look at, judge, censure, and denounce both ourselves as well as other people;

Experiential Avoidance
ACT is based on the assumption that the human language causes mental languishing unavoidably over us all. One way it does this is by setting us up to battle with our own considerations and sentiments, by methods for a procedure called experiential shirking.

The capacity to predict and solve problems was probably the single biggest evolutionary advantage in human language. This has not only allowed us to transform the face of the planet but also to fly outside it. This is the essence of problem-solving:
Problem= something we don't want.
Answer= find out or stop how to get rid of it.

Clearly this approach works well in the material world. A wolf standing outside your door? Get rid of this thing. Throw rocks or spears at him or shoot him. Snow, and rain, and hail? Okay, you cannot get out of this stuff, but by hiding in a hole or constructing a shelter, you can stop them. Dry, arid soil? Irrigation and fertilization will help you get rid of it, or you can stop it by moving to a better place. Consequently, critical thinking techniques are exceptionally versatile to us as people (and truth be told, instructing such abilities has demonstrated success in treating gloom). Given that this critical thinking approach functions admirably in the outside world, it's just normal for us to generally apply it to our internal world—the mental universe of contemplations, emotions, recollections, sensations and desires. Lamentably, very regularly, when we attempt to keep away from or free ourselves of undesirable private encounters, we're essentially making additional torment. For all intents and purposes, each enslavement referred to humanity starts as an endeavor to stay away from or dispose of undesirable contemplations and emotions, for example, weariness, forlornness, nervousness, sorrow, and so on. The addictive conduct at that point becomes self-continuing, as it gives a quick and simple approach to dispose of desires or side effects of withdrawal.

The more time and energy we expend trying to avoid or relieve ourselves of unwelcome private encounters, the more physically we are likely to suffer in the long run. Anxiety disorders are a good example of that. It is not the fear manifestation that constitutes the core of an anxiety disorder. Anxiety is a normal human emotion we all experience, after all. A major preoccupation with trying to avoid or get rid of anxiety is at the core of any anxiety disorder. OCD offers a florid example; I never cease to be amazed by the intricate routines invented by OCD sufferers, in futile efforts to get rid of thoughts and perceptions that cause anxiety. Sadly, the more importance we attach to avoiding anxiety, the more anxiety we develop over our anxiety— and this exacerbates it. It is a vicious cycle that is found at the heart of any anxiety disorder. (What is a fit of anxiety if not tension?) A huge assemblage of research shows that higher experiential evasion is related to uneasiness issues, despondency, more unfortunate work execution, more significant levels of substance misuse, lower personal satisfaction, high-chance sexual conduct, a marginal character issue, higher seriousness of PTSD, long haul inability and alexithymia.

Naturally, all forms of experiential avoidance are not unhealthy. Drinking a glass of wine to relax at night, for example, is experiential avoidance, but it is unlikely to be damaging. Yet consuming a whole bottle of wine a night would definitely be highly harmful in the long run. ACT often addresses experiential avoidance techniques when the customer employs them to such a degree that they become costly, life-distorting, or dangerous. ACT calls these "emotional control strategies" since they are attempts to control directly how we feel. A considerable lot of the passionate control methodologies that customers use to attempt to feel better (or feel "less terrible") may work for the time being. Nevertheless, they are regularly exorbitant and long haul pointless. Discouraged individuals, for instance, every now and again cease from associating to get away from meddling musings—"I'm a weight," "I don't have anything to do," "I'm not going to have a good time"—and negative feelings, for example, tension, weariness, and dread of dismissal. For the time being, dropping a social duty may offer ascent to a brief liberating sensation, however, the expanding social segregation will make them increasingly discouraged over the long haul.

Remedial INTERVENTIONS

ACT offers customers an option in contrast to experiential shirking through a scope of remedial intercessions. Customers, by and large, go to the treatment with a passionate control plan. They need to dispose of their downturn, uneasiness, drinking desires, horrendous recollections, low confidence, dismissal dread, outrage, despondency, and so on. There is no endeavor to lessen, change, maintain a strategic distance from, stifle, or control these private encounters inside ACT. Rather, by adequately utilizing care, customers figure out how to diminish the effect and impact of undesirable considerations and emotions. Customers figure out how to quit battling their private encounters—to open up to them, to prepare for them, and to permit them to go back and forth without a battle. The time, vitality, and cash recently squandered on attempting to control how they feel are then resources put into making powerful moves (guided by their qualities) to transform themselves to improve things.

Two key procedures depend on ACT mediations:

• Establishing information on unwelcome private collaborations that are out of close to home control

• Commitment to carrying on with an esteemed life, and activity

What follows is a brief overview of some middle ACT mediations, portrayed with vignettes of clinical work with a client named "Michael."
Going up against the Agenda

Right now, the passionate control plan of the customer is delicately and deferentially undermined by a procedure like persuasive talking.Clients describe forms they have tried to get rid of unwelcome private encounters or to stop them. You are then asked to assess for each method: "Will that in the long run each the symptoms? What's the expense of this approach in terms of time, money, fitness, resilience, relations? Has that got you back to the future that you want?"Michael was a 35-year-old bookkeeper who had incredible social nervousness and had seen various advisors futile. We went through the numerous systems he had utilized in the principal meeting to evade or dispose of his social uneasiness. They included: drinking liquor, taking Valium, being a "decent audience" (posing loads of inquiries, however sharing little of himself), showing up later than expected, leaving early, maintaining a strategic distance from get-togethers, by and large, breathing profoundly, loosening up procedures, utilizing positive attestations, contending negative musings, investigating his youth, accusing his folks (both of whom were socially abstaining from), instructing himself to "go over," Michael understood that none of those techniques had lessened his long haul tension. Albeit transient methodologies, for example, taking Valium, drinking liquor, and keeping away from get-togethers had diminished his tension, they had made considerable expenses to his personal satisfaction.His "primary work at home" was to see and record different procedures of passionate control and assess their long-haul viability and cost to his personal satisfaction.

Command is the problem, not the answer

In this process, we are that the perception of clients that emotional control techniques are largely responsible for their problems; that they are caught in a vicious cycle of growing misery as long as they are fixated on trying to control how they feel. Here appropriate examples like "quicksand," "war turn," "good discomfort," and "dirty discomfort" definitions. They might convey such metaphors like this: remember those old movies where the bad guy sinks into a swimming pool of quicksand, and the more he tries, the deeper he pulls him under? Struggling in quicksand is the worst you can possibly do. Lying back, stretching out your arms, and floating on the surface is the way to survive. It's tough because every instinct is urging you to fight; but if you do, you're going to drown.

The same principle applies to the feelings of difficulty: the more we try to fight them, the more they overwhelm us. Say that there is a "struggle light" at the back of our head. When it's turned on, it means that we're going to fight against any physical or emotional pain that comes our way; any stress we feel, we're going to try our hardest to get rid of it or stop it.

Suppose anxiety is the emotion that shows up. If our switch to fight is ON, then that feeling is totally unacceptable. It suggests that we could end up with frustration over our anxiety: "Why dare they make me feel this way?"Or sorrow over our anxiety:" Not again. How do I ever feel this way?"And panic for our anxiety:" What's wrong with me? What does this make for my body?"Or a blend of all these sentiments. These secondary emotions are useless, disagreeable and unhelpful, and a drain on our vitality. We get frustrated, nervous, or culpable in reaction. Look at that vicious cycle?

But what if our switch to combat is OFF? Whatever emotion shows up, we don't fight it, no matter how unpleasant it may be. So if there is fear, that's not a concern. Yeah, this is disagreeable. We don't like it, but it's nothing awful at the same moment. With the battle turn OFF, our level of anxiety is free to rise and fall as the situation dictates. These will sometimes be heavy, occasionally weak, and there will be no discomfort at all. Far more importantly, we don't waste our time and energy fighting against it.

We get a characteristic degree of physical and passionate uneasiness without battle, contingent upon what our identity is and in which circumstance we are in. We call this "perfect inconvenience" in ACT. We get a characteristic degree of physical and passionate distress without battle, contingent upon what our identity is and the circumstance we are in. In ACT, we term that "hot torment." There's no halting "warm distress." somehow, life offers it up to all of us.

When we begin to battle with it, be that as it may, our degrees of inconvenience increment quickly. We call this extra enduring "messy uneasiness." Our battle switch resembles a passionate enhancer — switch it on, and we may have displeasure regarding our tension, nervousness over our indignation, misery over our downturn, or blame over our blame.

Clearly, these allegories are custom-made to the specific sentiments with which the client battles. With the battle switch ON, we're not just sincerely upset by our own emotions, we're additionally doing all that we can to keep away from or dispose of them, paying little mind to the long-haul costs. We draw the consideration of customers to the numerous manners by which they have attempted to do this — through increasingly clear systems, for example, drugs, liquor, nourishment, TV, betting, smoking, sex, surfing the net — to less obvious passionate control procedures.For example, ruminating, chiding themselves, accusing others, and so on. (As referenced before, as long as they are utilized with some restraint, many control systems aren't an issue.) Michael had the option to effectively interface with these similitudes, particularly the possibility of a battle switch. In subsequent meetings, we had the option to allude back to that at whatever point he encountered uneasiness. "Alright, you're feeling on edge at the present time. Is the switch on or off of battle?"

Section 3

SIX CORE PRINCIPLES OF ACT

At that point, we present the six center standards of ACT once the passionate control motivation is undermined. ACT utilizes six center standards to assist customers with creating mental adaptability:

- Defusion

- Acceptance

- Contact with the present minute

- The Observing Self

- Values

- Committed Action

Every guideline has its own particular system, activities, schoolwork, and analogies. Take defusion, for example. Our considerations appear to be the exacting truth or decisions that must be complied, or huge occasions that require our complete consideration or compromising occasions that we need to dispose of. In different terms, they have a tremendous impact on our activities as we join with our feelings.

Cognitive defusion means that we can "step back" and watch language, without being caught in it. We should agree that our emotions are nothing more or less than fleeting private events— a constantly changing mix of phrases, sounds, and pictures. We have far less impact and influence because we defuse our emotions. Mental defusion ensures we will "step back" and analyze meaning, without being trapped in it. We should agree that our emotions are nothing more or less than fleeting private events— a constantly changing mix of phrases, sounds, and pictures. They have far less impact and influence as we defuse our thoughts.

Going through the wide variety of ACT publications, you'll discover about a hundred different techniques of temporal defusion. For example, to manage an upsetting idea, we may very well watch it with separation; or rehash it again and again, out loud, until it just turns into an unimportant sound; or envision it in an animation character's voice; or sing it in the tune of "Upbeat Birthday;" or quietly state "Much appreciated, mind" in appreciation for such an intriguing idea. There will never be less space for a creative mind. Like CBT, not one of those strategies in intellectual defusion incorporates investigating or contesting undesirable musings.

Here's a simple exercise for yourself in cognitive defusion:

Step 1: Recall an upsetting and recurring negative self-judgment that takes the form of "I am X," such as

"I am incompetent," or "I am stupid." Hold that idea in your psyche for a couple of moments and trust it as much as you can. Presently notice the effect it has on you.

Stage 2: Now take the idea "I am X" and add this expression before it: "I have the idea that...." Now run that while reconsidering the new expression this time around. If you don't mind, note what happens.

In stage two, the vast majority notice a "separation" from the idea, so it has far less impact. Notice that no exertion has been made to dispose of the idea, nor transform it. Or maybe the association with the reasoning has changed — it must be viewed as expressions.

CHAPTER 3

A CONCISE DEPICTION OR THE SIX CENTER STANDARDS FOLLOWS HERE, REGARDING THE CASE OR MICHAEL

1. Psychological Defusion: figuring out how to see contemplations, pictures, recollections and different comprehensions as what they seem to be—just bits of language, words, and pictures—rather than what they may give off an impression of being—undermining occasions, decisions that must be complied, target certainties and realities.

During meeting two, Michael said he felt intermittent nervousness from sentiments, including "I'm dull," "I don't have anything to tell," "Nobody likes me," and "I'm a washout." As the meeting advanced, I helped Michael manage these musings in various manners before they started to lose impact. First of all, I caused him to bring the reasoning "I am a washout" to mind. At that point, he shut his eyes and considered where it was by all accounts in space. He detected it was in front of him. I requested that he watch the idea as though he were an inquisitive researcher, and to see its state: regardless of whether it was progressively similar to something that he could see or hear. He said it resembled words he could see, and he saw it turned out to be less troubling as he "looked" at it. I asked him to imagine the thought as words on a

Karaoke screen; then change the font; then change the colour; then imagine a bouncing ball jumping from word to word. I asked him to imagine the thought as words on a Karaoke screen; then change the font; then change the color; then imagine a bouncing ball jumping from word to word. By this time, Michael was chuckling at the very same idea that he had been brought to tears just a few minutes earlier. "Homework" involved learning many different techniques of defusion for distressing thoughts— not to get rid of them but merely to know how to step back and see them for what they are — just going by "parts of words."

2. Acknowledgment: accounting for undesirable sentiments, sensations, inclinations, and other private encounters, permitting them to go back and forth without battling with them, run from them, or give them undue consideration.

I asked Michael, in meeting three, to get on edge by envisioning himself at a pending office party. He revealed a "monster tie" in his stomach when I requested that he examine his body and notice where he felt the tension most seriously. I instructed him to examine this wonder as though he were a youthful researcher who had never observed anything like it; to note its outlines, its form, its vibration, its weight, its temperature, its pulsation, and the multitude of other sensations within the sensation. I made him relax into the feeling, to "make room for it;" to let it be there, even if he didn't like it or needed it. Eventually, Michael mentioned a sense of calm, a sensation of being at home with his fear even though he didn't like that. With his repetitive sentiments of uneasiness, "Schoolwork" included rehearsing this method—not to dispose of them, however basically to figure out how to allow them to travel every which way without a battle.

3. Contact the present minute: carrying full attention to your experience here-and-now, with receptiveness, intrigue, and receptivity; concentrating on and completely captivating in whatever you do.
I brought Michael through a basic relaxation practice in session four, based on the eating experience. I presented to him a sultana and requested that he eat it "in moderate movement," with a complete spotlight on the natural product's taste and surface, and on the sounds, sensations, and developments inside his mouth.I let him know, "While you're doing this, there may come up a wide range of diverting considerations and sentiments. The objective is just to allow your considerations to go back and forth and let your emotions be there, and keep your consideration concentrated on eating the sultana. "Michael subsequently said he was amazed that there was so much flavor in a single sultan. Then I was able to use this insight to draw an analogy with social situations where Michael was so caught up with his thoughts and feelings that he couldn't completely engage in conversation, so lost out on "richness." "Homework"

involved exercising full involvement with all five senses in a number of daily activities (dushing, brushing his teeth, and cleaning his dishes) as if it were a matter of recourse. He even promised to exercise constructive participation in conversations; i.e., to hold his focus to the other person, rather than his own thoughts and feelings.

4. The Observing Self: getting to a powerful sentiment of self, an intelligence of mindfulness that is interminable, ever-present, and harmless.From this viewpoint, you can legitimately encounter not consider, emotions, recollections, urges, sensations, pictures, jobs, or physical body. These wonders are continually changing and fringe parts of you, yet they are not the quintessence of what your identity is. The Observing Self: access to an extraordinary feeling of self, a constant, ever-present, and innocuous congruity of cognizance.

I took Michael through a care practice in meeting five intended to have him able to access that extraordinary self. Next, I guided him to close his eyes and look at his contemplations: the shape they were rolling, their undeniable situation in space, the force they were going at. At that point, I solicited him: "Be aware of what you see. The emotions are there ,and you note them. So there are two procedures going on —a manner of thinking, and a procedure of seeing that reasoning." Over and over, I caused him to notice the differentiation between the contemplations that emerge and the self that watches those considerations. Any reasoning is destructive, harming, or controlling, from the Observing Self perspective.

5. Values: clarifying what's most important, deep within your heart; what kind of person you want to be; what's meaningful to you; and what you want to stand for in this life.

Michael established important values in session six about communicating with others, creating meaningful friendships, cultivating trust, and being sincere and real. We discussed the Willingness concept. The willingness to feel anxiety does not mean that you want it or do not like it. Instead it means that you allow it to be there to do something that you value. I asked Michael, "If taking your life toward these values means that you need to make room for anxious feelings, are you willing to do that?"His answer was, yea."

6. Committed action: to set goals, to guide your values, and to take effective action to reach them.
Continuing the sixth session, we shifted to set goals according to Michael's principles. At first, he set the objective of eating day by day with a partner grinding away and sharing some close to home data on each event. He set out, continuously testing social targets in gatherings and continued practicing care aptitudes to manage the tense contemplations and feelings that would develop. Michael announced toward the finish

of ten meetings that he was mingling substantially more, and all the more significantly, that he was getting a charge out of it. Considerations of being "a failure" or "exhausting" or "unlikeable" frequently existed, yet he didn't, for the most part, pay attention to them or give any consideration to them.Similarly, in many social situations, feelings of anxiety still occurred but no longer bothered him or distracted him. Generally, his levels of anxiety have significantly diminished. The decrease of fear was not a treatment goal but a fun by-product.

It shows how ACT will lead to a good reduction of symptoms without ever reaching for it. First, there was a lot of exposure, as Michael was engaged in ever more challenging social situations. Exposure is well known to often contribute to decreased distress. Additionally, the more tolerant Michael became of his unwelcome thoughts and feelings, the less distress he had over those feelings and thoughts. In fact, the practice of mindfulness of unwanted thoughts and feelings is in itself a form of exposure.

THE TRAINING OF ACT THERAPEUTIC RELATIONSHIP

ACT assists advisors with building up the basic characteristics of sympathy, acknowledgment, compassion, regard, and the capacity to remain mentally present even among forceful feelings. Also, ACT instructs specialists that they are in a similar vessel as their customers, on account of human language—so they should be illuminated creatures or "have everything in perfect order." Indeed, they may state something as: "I don't need you to think I have my life all together. It's progressively similar to your ascending your mountain over yonder, and here I'm ascending my mountain. It's not as if I found a good pace, and I'm having a rest. It's simply that I can see obstructions on your mountain from where I'm on my mountain which you can't see. So I can point those out to you, and maybe give you some elective courses around them.

With ACT, the experience of undergoing the treatment is immeasurably unique. It's not tied in with disposing of awful sentiments or traversing old injury anymore. Rather it is tied in with making a rich, significant, and full life. This is supported by the results of Strosahl, Hayes, Bergan, and Romano7, who have shown that ACT improves therapy effectiveness and Hayes et al. (2004), who have shown that burnout decreases. If I had to sum up ACT on a t-shirt, it would read: "Embrace your demon, and follow your heart."

ACT'S ABCS — ACCEPTANCE AND COMMITMENT THERAPY

This subtle verbal and cognitive shift is the essence of acceptance and commitment therapy (ACT). This indicates a person can take action without modifying or withdrawing emotions first. Instead of fighting the feeling attached to behavior, a person can look at himself as having the feeling but still acting. Acceptance-based strategies postulate that the most effective approach may be to accept and improve rather than to aim for improvement alone. In the Serenity Prayer, the importance of acceptance was long recognized.

ACT is being assessed as one of the postmodern conduct approaches as another momentary intercession in an assortment of populaces saw by social laborers.

Evolution in ACT

Psychodynamic methods that promote intuition means that most certainly a change of attitude would result in a change in actions. Pure behavioral approaches, by contrast, suggest that altering behavior does not require a change of attitude. Changing behavior can, however, eventually lead to a change in attitude or emotion. The focus is on changing behavior of whatever underlying emotion.

Taking behaviorism a step further, ACT suggests that simultaneous and independent behavior and emotion can exist. Acceptance has been described as the "traditional behavior therapy missing link."ACT is a piece of more extensive development in the conduct and psychological domains that incorporates the ways to deal with care.

Hayes was credited with being ACT's author as a logical way to deal with treatment. He investigates setting mysteries, for example, isolating words and activities, and recognizing the feeling of self of the customers from their considerations and conduct. For example, if an individual doesn't go to work since the person in question is on edge about an encounter with their chief, it is possible (and empowered) that the individual can go to work while feeling on edge. A significant objective of treatment is to show customers that they can live with nervousness and dispose of the control that settings apply. Those acquainted with objective passionate conduct treatment will perceive this methodology as steady with ("orders") oral administration of rules.

ACT is conceived of the treatment school of conduct. Social treatment, be that as it may, is partitioned into three ages: conventional behavioralism, psychological conduct treatment (CBT), and current "third era" or relevant conduct draws near. This third influx of behaviorism has an existential twist in its reason that enduring is a key trait of human life and speaks to an emotional change from conventional behaviorism and CBT because of the incorporation of acknowledgment and care based mediations. The third wave, which likewise incorporates argumentative social treatment and subjective treatment dependent on care, causes to notice the mental, relevant and experiential universe of its constituents.

The conviction behind ACT is that defeating negative contemplations and sentiments can accomplish a progressively satisfying life. ACT's point is to help customers reliably decide to act adequately (solid practices as characterized by their qualities) within sight of "private" (subjective or mental) occasions that are troublesome or problematic. Regularly, the term ACT was utilized to depict what occurs in treatment: perceive the outcomes of the hardships of life, select persuading standards, and make a move.

Hypothetical Base

Writing about ACT is restricted in social work. As is run of the mill of a significant part of the subordinate information base of social work, writing from the fields of brain research and social brain science adds to getting ACT and its application to the act of social work. The ACT writing goes back to the mid-1980s yet has, all the more as of late, indicated logical potential.

ACT is an extraordinary psychotherapeutic strategy dependent on the hypothesis of association outlines (RFT). RFT questions the setting wherein procedures for objective change exist, in view of social examination standards. RFT gives a comprehension of the intensity of verbal conduct and language by looking at the association's individuals have with their regular and social conditions (settings). The hypothesis holds that quite a bit of what we term psychopathology is the aftereffect of the human propensity to evade private occasions that are antagonistically evaluated (what we think and feel). ACT represents the structures where jargon powers individuals into endeavors to take up arms against their internal life. Customers figure out how to recontextualize and acknowledge these private occasions, create more noteworthy clearness about close to home estimations, and focus on the necessary change in conduct. This hypothesis is best comprehended for social laborers as "individual in world," with the extra component of how jargon is utilized to see and explore certain circumstances.

Procedure

The center of ACT is a change in verbal conduct both inside (self-talk) and outside (activity). It is liberating to simply watch oneself with emotions and to perceive and acknowledge that sentiments are a characteristic outgrowth of conditions. Customers have feelings in regards to their affections (first of all, they may be humiliated to be discouraged, irate, or miserable). ACT says they deteriorate off fighting emotions. "On the off chance that you can't acknowledge the inclination for the present, you'll be left with it, yet on the off chance that you can, you can change your reality so you won't have that feeling later." It clarifies that ACT doesn't mean we request that customers acknowledge each circumstance (for example, damaging connections) yet that a few conditions ought to, at last, be acknowledged (e.g., physical reality or chronicled occasions).

For instance, if a customer is upset by recollections of past occasions, the person needs to acknowledge that the occasion happened; may in the long run, decrease going with emotions. This idea is suggestive of the point of view of the qualities of social work, in which Saleebey exhorts that the decision can be acknowledged at this point oppose the sentence.

Mattaini, a suggestive of the Serenity Prayer, alerts that the underlying work is to distinguish zones that can and can not be changed. Physical handicaps and past injury are instances of things that can not and are best acknowledged.
ACT focuses on shifting from the experiential content to the experience context. Hayes describes six core ACT processes: acceptance, cognitive defusion, presence, self as context, appreciation, and committed action. Likewise, a sample model for intervention is provided by Wilson and his colleagues. Clients often have a goal of eradicating the past or the pain associated with that. They struggled with "the problem" in many different ways for a long time. Thus, evasive behaviors are assessed initially. What was the "experiential resistance" to the client?—that which happens when an individual is unable to remain in contact with specific private interactions and takes steps to change the type or duration of those

incidents and the circumstances that induce them, even when doing so causes psychological damage.

2. Examine those strategies that didn't work. The paradox is that having to work hard to solve the problem makes the problem appear worse. ACT views the problem-solving method rationale as faulty because it is focused on historically accepted, language-based guidelines for problem-solving. Such laws are taken for granted, as an alternative to a psychological problem is the existence of negative inward perceptions (feelings, emotions, sensations). Getting safe then, by extension, implies avoiding these negative experiences. The ACT advisor is attempting to challenge these principles by exhibiting that endeavors dependent on these guidelines can, in actuality, be the wellspring of issues. An increasingly legitimate and solid wellspring of critical thinking is simply the immediate experience of the customer and their input from life. "It isn't the life of the individual which is sad, nor experiential administration (shirking) strategies which are sad."

3. Set up power with contrasting strategies. A lifetime of diverting oneself from aversive private encounters is similar to fleeing from one's shadow constantly. The result is that one is at a misfortune for balance in other life circumstances by endeavoring to control the damaging musings and sentiments.

4. Recognize that self as setting, recognized in content from self, is like the way toward externalizing account ways to deal with the issue. Customers are encouraged to come into contact with an attentive self—the person who is continually watching and seeing is not the same as one's own discernment.

5. Powerlessness to be socially flexible might be supported by a misconception of standards or a crisscross of objectives with convictions. Therefore, the following stage in the ACT procedure is to "pick a heading and set up readiness" and to distinguish inspiring qualities and build up an eagerness to help recapture control of life, not really just to control musings and emotions. Ability is neither renunciation, nor is it equivalent to want. It is an ability to encounter, acknowledge, and face "negative enthusiastic states evaluated. Once more, the distinction between being willing and feeling willing is noted. The model given is that you probably won't feel all set to the dental specialist, yet you may have the option to go at any rate.

6. Duty in the last phases of treatment is the core interest. The dedication is to surrender the war of dismissing or battling one's past and enthusiastic states to discover open doors for social control.

Techniques

Frequently used with ACT, diagrams, paradoxes, and experiential experiments. Many interventions are smart, creative, and playful. ACT procedures can vary from brief, in-minute measures to those that cover several hours. Under the following five guidelines, there are various methods listed which are extrapolated from the therapeutic resources gathered by Gifford, Hayes, and Stroshal; this on record was found to take place in 2005. These constitute only a fraction of the material available to clinicians as resources.

1.   Facing the current situation ("creative hopelessness") encourages clients to see what they've tried to do better, examine whether they've really worked, and create space for something new to occur. Facing the unworkable truth of their numerous encounters frequently leaves the client in a condition of "imaginative sadness," not recognizing what to do straightaway. The state is innovative in light of the fact that totally new methodologies can be created without utilizing the past standards administering their conduct.

2. Acknowledgment procedures are intended to lessen the inspiration expected to maintain a strategic distance from specific circumstances. "Unfastening" is given an accentuation—understanding that musings and emotions don't generally prompt activities. These systems are regularly done "in vivo," which structures meeting encounters. It is a notable concentration to separate between considerations, sentiments, and encounters.

3. The deliteralization of psychological defusion reclassifies thinking and encountering as a progressing procedure of conduct, not a result. Strategies are proposed to show that considerations are only musings and not really real factors. It can include sitting alongside the customer, advancing each idea and experience as an article with an end goal to "defuse and deliteralize."

4. Esteeming as a decision explains what the client esteems for the wellbeing of its own: What offers importance to life? The objective is to assist customers with understanding the qualification between a worth and an objective, pick their qualities and announce them, and set social errands related with to qualities.

5. Self as setting shows the customer to consider his to be her way of life as unmistakable from the substance of their experience.

Potential ACT populaces have been exactly tried, and there is motivation to accept that an assortment of populaces could profit by this. Fundamental research showed that ACT is valuable for overcomers of sexual maltreatment, youths in danger, and those with substance misuse or mindset issue. It was recommended in 2005 by Hayes that the ACT model appears to work over a bizarrely wide exhibit of issues.

ACT would be appropriate for individuals with substance misuse issues, through positive training and improvement methodologies. With those encountering insane ideation, ACT has been utilized. For one survey, mental patients with ACT demonstrated improvement for full of feeling manifestations, psychological brokenness, and pipedream related nervousness.

For injury work, just as for those with fears and over the top conduct, ACT was proposed. It appears to be especially important to utilize ACT approaches with injury exploited people. The individuals who experience the ill effects of posttraumatic stress may profit by tolerating the experience without surrendering to their residuals. The hesitance to encounter injury-related agony makes an inner battle (verbal fight) that keeps the injury alive.

ACT might be a powerful device for social specialists managing youth misuse survivors. The comprehensions and sentiments emerging from a background marked by misuse are inclined to transform from an ACT perspective. CBT might be hoping to change oneself talk structure. On the other hand, ACT tries to change the job of contemplations and emotions. As far as their sensible sensibility, intellectual treatment thinks about negative musings and emotions; ACT centers around their mental sensibility. It isn't particularly useful to tell an unfortunate interbreedingcasualty that her irritating feelings are unwarranted in conditions of sexual closeness. The mental capacity of those considerations is progressively helpful to bring up.

ACT has been proposed for couples and families to work with. One investigation indicated that agreeableness procedures expanded the viability of conventional conjugal social treatment. The objective isn't to acknowledge all accomplice practices essentially however, to viably "produce a setting wherein both acknowledgment and change will happen". Three manners by which ACT intercessions assist couples with creating more noteworthy closeness with the zone of contention utilized as a vehicle, produce resilience, and achieve change. Acknowledgment isn't recognizing the activities of another, nor relinquishing the battle to attempt to change the direction of another.

Obviously, preparation is recommended for being qualified as an ACT teacher. ACT has a place for social workers dealing with a wide range of behavioral problems that require short and empirically based intervention. "Get off your goals" is one of the techniques used in ACT, where all the "buts" are replaced by "and." So instead of saying, "I'd like to learn about ACT but don't have the time," consider saying, "I'd like to learn about ACT, and it's worth the time!"

THE ROLE OF ACT IN PSYCHOLOGY AND MINDFULNESS

Acceptance and Commitment Therapy is based on Relational Framework Theory, a theory based on the idea that human capacity to relate is the basis for language and cognition.

Relating involves noting the dimensions the relationship exists alongside. We might be partner an apple with an orange, for instance, however our capacity to relate permits us to get that despite the fact that they have a comparable shape (round) and work (to be eaten), they have various hues and surfaces.

In contrast with most different species, the job of ACT in brain science and care has an unimaginable capacity to relate to even ominous things, just as apparently inconsequential terms and ideas.

While this is a profitable capacity, it likewise encourages negative contemplations and self-judgment. On the off chance that we can relate "treat" to the treat eating experience, at that point, we can likewise relate "useless" to feeling we're useless.

The capacity to frame correspondence systems (e.g., I associate the expressions "green," "apple," and "pear" to the meaning of "organic product") can be an adverse ability as nervousness and gloom sway us.

For example, we may relate "useless" to a capacity to play out my activity and relate "useless" to my life by expansion. ACT depends on the Theory of Relational Blocks.

We regularly make relationship arrangements that are not complimentary or nurturing, yet we can likewise change those connections in the event that we apply attention to acknowledge our sentiments and change how we respond and identify with them, rather than endeavoring to avoid them.

CHAPTER 4

Clinical APPLICATION OF ACT IN TREATING LIFE THREATENING CONDITIONS

TREATING DEPRESSION WITH ACT

Acknowledgment and Commitment Therapy (ACT) is another type of intellectual, social treatment (CBT) that has increased more consideration as of late. It looks at how the communication between the musings, emotions, and conduct of an individual affects prosperity and afterward assists with changing the association to deliver more prominent fulfillment throughout everyday life. Within sight of difficult musings and sentiments, ACT utilizes practices of care to assist individuals with expanding mindfulness and build up a mentality of acknowledgment and empathy. What's more, ACT emphatically focuses on the job of qualities in helping individuals make important lives. ACT assists individuals with bypassing perception in those everyday issues where it is less helpful and the psyche may have created restricting principles and assists individuals with strengthening parts of discernment where it will be generally helpful, for example, in resolving to esteemed living.

ACT is especially useful in taking care of burdensome sentiments as it gives individuals an approach to building up another relationship with agony and languishing.A fundamental assumption of ACT is that pain is a normal and inevitable part of human experience and that having whatever emotions arise in the presence of painful experiences is perfectly healthy. Nevertheless, the natural tendency of individuals to regulate or prevent their own thoughts and feelings can in fact lead to much long-term and unnecessary suffering. For example, an individual can create short-term ways to cope with their feelings—such as social withdrawal, drug usage, or over-consumption—that actually end up causing even more long-term misery. Worse yet, time spent struggling with thoughts and feelings is a time away from life's most important things. Simply put, ACT is about letting go of the struggle with hard thoughts and feelings to pursue a richer, fuller, and more purposive life.

Acceptance and commitment therapy is a psychotherapy that is based on evidence. Its practitioners and researchers are dedicated to the therapy's scientific development and empirical evaluation of its impacts. ACT was evaluated in over 300 randomized clinical trials and proved helpful in addressing a wide range of mental health concerns. Moreover, ACT has been demonstrated to be as compelling in improving moderate to extreme wretchedness levels as Cognitive Therapy–the present highest quality level psychotherapy.

ACT Is a Little-Known, Fast Depression Treatment Some analysts accept that tolerating your negative contemplations can assist them with overcoming all the more rapidly.

Scott Stambach felt devoured by nervousness, in some cases to the point of wheezing for breath, at whatever point he needed to stand up out in the open —an especially extraordinary issue for a person who was preparing to be an educator. It just exacerbated the situation by battling his feelings of trepidation, which would rise even days before he needed to give a talk. At that point, he unearthed a book that upheld a more chill approach: watching his evil presences and tolerating them as opposed to attempting to wreck them.

"The thought that I could stop the war I was having with myself gave me a colossal positive feeling," Stambach, presently a 37-year-old secondary school and junior college instructor in San Diego, lets me know. "You can prepare for that dread, even love it. This has completely changed me." While ACT was made in the 1980s, adequate investigations have been led to give it more extensive road credits just as of late. Proof has now indicated that ACT is successful in treating nervousness, sleep deprivation, interminable agony, and habit, among different clutters, despite the fact that there are numerous little investigations.

ACT is a type of subjective conduct treatment (CBT). In any case, while an advisor will urge you to challenge yourself in exemplary CBT and attempt to change your negative or unreasonable considerations, ACT needs you to be increasingly careful and acknowledge them. Another research paper published in 2015 in Psychotherapy and Psychomatics contrasted the two approaches, finding that ACT tends to be more effective in treating various mental health conditions, although the writers do suggest that more studies are needed.

"At the moment when you meditate, you let your thoughts go through like a cloud in the sky, noticing them instead of pushing them away. ACT is based on this idea," explains Steven C. Hayes, a professor of psychology at the University of Nevada and a founder of the method. What's key here, he says, isn't cleaning up your thoughts, "it's changing your relationship with the world within you." Determining what's important to you (i.e., your values) is another part of the therapy. "It's important for you to ask yourself what kind of life you want to live on once you stop fighting your thoughts," says Hayes, who wrote the 2005 seminal book on ACT, Get Out of Your Mind and Into Your Life.

The ways in which you get to that detached state, or in ACT-speaking, "defused" state, where you see those thoughts simply as flickers in your brain waves, may seem strange at first. You can sing the thought, a favored Stambach technique ("I'm going to panic in front of everyone," he'd croon, which makes it seem less serious); distill it to a single word and repeat it for 30 seconds ("faint, faint, faint"). One woman who discovered ACT for her eating disorder in a recovery program found it helpful to say, "I'm noticing that I'm thinking I'm feeling anxious," which made it less overwhelming than her previous lament, "I'm anxious." Isolating the issue from the feeling can change your whole experience of this, says Megan Call, a clinical therapist who uses ACT with University customers. After a long run, an elite runner may experience the same pain as someone with a physical disability, she observes, but the runner does not believe that he will be limited by the pain, nor does the person with the disability. "There's a distinction between saying,' I can't handle this scenario,' versus' I'm afraid I can't handle it,'" explains Call. The latter could cause you to know that you can indeed.

Jonathan Bricker, an associate professor of psychology at the University of Washington, explains how he began to see that ACT is more successful at managing cravings such as junk food or nicotine than the typical approach to attempting to gin up willpower. With a starving beast, you can not win a tug-of-war, he says in the conversation, because the monster will eventually win and you will give in. ACT lets you drop the rope. "If you just let the monster occupy a space in your body, you'll discover that [he] isn't as threatening as he appears to be, and sometimes he even goes away," Bricker notes.

The method, of course, has its critics. Some researchers believe the evidence is not yet strong enough to give up on long-used treatments, particularly for complex conditions such as obsessive-compulsive disorder. Others note that in your everyday life, you have to remember to use the tools, which can be challenging since the techniques are hardly intuitive. One depressed man admits he has forgotten, over time, to "defuse" his thoughts, leading to his depression returning.

The good thing about ACT is that it is considered, like CBT, to be successful after just a couple of meetings, not the years of appointments other forms of treatment need. If your insurance coverage covers mental health, it should include ACT courses. A therapist can be found in your area on Psychology Today's or the Contextual Behavioral Science Association websites. Research has shown you can also benefit from working online with a therapist or using workbooks, as has Stambach.

Stambach concedes in the years since finding that book that he still, in some cases, feels apprehensive when remaining before a gathering. Be that as it may, presently, he realizes he shouldn't pay attention to those apprehensions so."My mind had previously treated anxious thoughts as the gospel, and now I have a far more playful relationship with them," he says.

A New Approach to Depression Treatment

Acceptance and Commitment Therapy, or ACT, is a' modern generation' approach to dealing with a range of psychiatric problems and treatment for depression. While ACT is moderately new contrasted with all the more regularly rehearsed approaches, it has been utilized and read for a very long while by clinicians, and there is a lot of logical proof to recommend that it is effective at achieving positive changes in the lives of customers.

What constitutes depression?

A person may be depressed if he or she experiences five or more of the following difficulties over a period of two weeks that significantly impair daily functioning: low mood for most of the day, significantly less interest or pleasure in most or all of the activities that he or she usually enjoys.

Twenty percent of Australian women and roughly 13 percent of Australian men will experience depression during their lifetime, according to Beyond Blue.

How is one diagnosed with depression?
If you believe you may experience depression, it's important to discuss your difficulties with your GP. The GP should conduct an extensive medical exam to ensure that the symptoms are not caused by another health problem. For further assessment and treatment, the doctor may refer you to a mental health specialist, such as a psychologist.

What exactly is ACT?

ACT involves the practice of a conscious awareness of positive, neutral, and negative experiences, both internal (feelings and thoughts) and external (behaviors and stimuli to the environment).

This awareness is used to facilitate' defusion'–the practice of creating space between those experiences and the self. Many anxious people ' fuse' with disturbing emotions (e.g., 'I am a failure') and perceptions (e.g., hopelessness), which then stops them from engaging in activities that they normally enjoy or contribute to a positive existence (e.g., meeting friends regularly, working out).

The creation of space allows customers to place less emphasis on upsetting thoughts, feelings, and situations that facilitate engagement in a more valued life. When a troubled person may see that they are not their thoughts and feelings, they are more likely to choose to behave according to their beliefs, rather than asking them what their mind or body thinks.

How does ACT vary from other strategies to treat depression?
Some other styles of psychological therapy involve training in skills to assess the rationality of negative thoughts and feelings and developing more realistic styles of thinking. While these abilities can also be quite useful, it is unrealistic to expect people to always be able to think rationally, and sometimes human negative thoughts and feelings are perfectly realistic and relevant to the situation in question.

Of starters, a frustrated person with chronic pain will believe that' I'm never going to be well again'-this may really be a rational idea. A rational assessment of it is unlikely to help a person feel more positive and have a happier and more meaningful life. Nevertheless, it is often more rewarding to encourage the client to understand that they can have the feeling, and still engage in meaningful and rich experiences (e.g., visiting a friend).

Medication is also a growing approach to treating depression. This is appropriate in many cases, as some people experience such a low mood that they are unable to motivate themselves to do just about anything. Medication can be a useful first step in facilitating engagement with treatment in more severe cases. Nonetheless, depression almost always develops by combining biological, psychological, and social factors. If treatment is used in combination with psychiatric therapy, only part of the problem is resolved, and it's impossible to have a complete recovery.

TREATMENT OF POST-TRAUMATIC STRESS DISORDER WITH ACT

Post-traumatic stress disorder can occur to a person following a traumatic event that caused them to feel frightened, surprised, or powerless. It can have long-term effects, including nightmares, breathing problems, and anxiety.

Types of incidents that may cause post-traumatic stress disorder (PTSD) involve battles, murders, explosions, injuries, a loved one's death, or some form of abuse. Thoughts and memories recur even if the hazard has passed.

About seven and eight percent of the population is believed to be impaired, although women are more likely to be impacted than men.

The patient may become more nervous and afraid instead of getting better as time goes by. Over the years, PTSD may interrupt a person's life, however, therapy may help them recover.

Side effects and indications of the analysis generally start inside three months of an occasion, yet can start later.

For an individual to be determined to have PTSD, they should meet the criteria set out in the Fifth Edition of the Diagnostic and Statistical Manual of the American Psychological Association (APA) (DSM-5).

Those rules require the individual to:

1. Have been presented to death or undermined with death, genuine injury or sexual savagery, regardless of whether legitimately, by seeing it, through happening to a friend or family member, or during proficient obligations

2. Experience the following for more than a month:
   - one or more intrusion symptoms
   - one or more withdrawal symptoms
   - two or more symptoms influencing attitude and thought
   - two or more anxiety and reactivity symptoms that begin after the incident

Here are some descriptions of these four forms of symptoms:

Intrusion symptoms: memories of the dreams and a sense that the occurrence is occurring again.

Fearful thoughts Avoid symptoms: refuse to discuss the event avoiding situations that remind the person of the event Arousal and reactivity symptoms: difficulty sleeping irritability and angry outbursts hypersensitivity to possible hazards feeling tense what's more, on edge side effects influencing disposition and thinking: failure to recollect certain parts of the occasion sentiments of blame and accused.

Physical side effects

Physical indications may likewise happen, yet these are excluded from the DSM-5 criteria: physical impacts that incorporate perspiring, shaking, migraines, discombobulation, stomach issues, a throbbing painfulness, and chest torment a debilitated safe framework can prompt increasingly visit rest unsettling influences that can prompt weariness and different issues. The individual may start devouring more liquor than previously or may abuse medications or prescriptions.
Children and adolescents.In those six years old or under, side effects may include: bedwetting subsequent to figuring out how to utilize the restroom, the kid might not have flashbacks and might not experience issues recalling portions of the occasion when playing with a grown-up. They may review it in an alternate request, however, or feel there was an indication that it would occur.

They may likewise have the option to carry on or express the injury through play, pictures, and stories. We may have mind flights, and they may get crabby. They may think that it's hard to go to class, or to invest energy with companions or considering.

Youngsters by and large will, in general, show comparative responses to grown-ups from age eight or more.

The individual can show problematic or insolent, hasty, or forceful conduct between the ages of 12 and 18.

They may feel remorseful through the span of the occasion for not acting contrastingly or they may think about retribution.

Kids who have encountered sexual maltreatment are bound to: feel dread, pity, uneasiness, and seclusion. They also may have a low feeling of self-esteem, conduct themselves in a forceful way, showing bizarre sexual conduct, and harming themselves. Medication or liquor screening may be conducted. As a component of the symptomatic procedure, the individual might be given a screening test to survey whether they have PTSD or not.

The time taken for this may differ between 15 minutes and a few one-hour meetings. In the event that there are lawful ramifications, or if a handicap guarantee relies upon it, a more extended evaluation might be utilized.

On the off chance that the manifestations vanish following half a month, intense pressure issue might be analyzed.

PTSD will in general last more, with progressively serious manifestations and may not show up until some time after the occasion.

Numerous individuals recoup inside a half year, however for quite a long while, some are as yet encountering side effects.

Causes

Some people experience PTSD when returning from conflict zones.
PTSD may develop following a traumatic occurrence.

Examples include:
- military confrontation
- natural disasters
- serious accidents
- terrorist attack
- loss of a loved one, whether or not this involves violence
- rape or other types of personal abuse being a victim of crime receiving a life-threatening diagnosis

Any circumstance that triggers dread, stun, repulsiveness or weakness can prompt PTSD.

Hazard factors

Where a few people create PTSD, it stays indistinct why others don't. In any case, the accompanying danger variables may improve the probability of encountering indications: having extra issues after an occasion. For instance, losing a friend or family member and losing an employment without social help after an occasion with a background marked by emotional wellness issues or exploiting past understanding of misuse previously or because of an occasion during youth. These can possibly affect dread, misery, and PTSD.

Mind structure: Brain examinations indicated that, contrasted with others, the hippocampus seems diverse in individuals with PTSD. The hippocampus is associated with handling feelings and recollections, and it could influence the opportunity of having flashbacks.

Reaction to push: levels of hormones typically discharged in a battle or-flight circumstance in individuals with PTSD seem, by all accounts, to appear as something else.

Sexual orientation: This can have a section to play. Studies propose that while men are bound to encounter brutality, females are bound to have PTSD.

What are the components that bring down the hazard?

Researchers are taking a gander at variables of versatility that may assist individuals with recuperating all the more successfully from or maintain a strategic distance from PTSD.

These include:

having or looking for help from others with or creating adapting procedures the capacity of the individual to like how they act when confronted with trouble. When seeing a specialist, Many individuals experience manifestations following an awful mishap, for example, crying, nervousness, and focus trouble, yet this isn't really PTSD.

Brief consideration with an expert professional can assist with keeping the indications from deteriorating.

This ought to be considered if: side effects endure for manifestations that are extreme enough for over a month to keep the individual from coming back to typical life that the individual considers hurting themselves.

These include: work trouble or associations with a higher danger of heart issues, a higher possibility of constant illness, the chance of changes influencing the cerebrum, including more elevated levels of the pressure hormone cortisol, and abatement in the size of the hippocampus–a mind structure that is significant in memory handling and feeling.

Counteraction: can it?

Individuals who work in callings where awful accidents like the military and crisis administrations are probably going to happen can be offered preparation or guidance to assist them with adapting to or diminish the danger of PTSD.

A kind of questioning known as Critical Incident Stress Management (CISM) happens after specific episodes in the crisis clinical administrations (EMS) so as to attempt to limit the danger of stress and creating PTSD.

The efficacy of this has been debated, however, and some studies have suggested it may be detrimental, as it may interfere with the normal recovery process, for example, by pressuring people to face memories and emotions before they are able to do so.

CHAPTER 5

ACCEPTANCE AND COMMITMENT THERAPY (ACT) FOR PTSD

A number of people have been successful in using posttraumatic stress disorder (PTSD) acceptance and committed therapy (ACT). If you are dealing with PTSD symptoms, ACT may be effective with PTSD. Realize why this treatment can help and what the five treatment objectives are.

The Rationale Behind Acceptance and Commitment Therapy for PTSD

We figured out how to name emotions as awful and others as great since the beginning. Bitterness and trouble, for instance, are seen as acceptable or hopeful sentiments and joy and satisfaction as awful or negative.

It's reasonable, at that point, that we attempt to have however many agonizing sentiments as could be expected under the circumstances, and the same number of positive ones. Particularly when we feel enthusiastic agony, we will, in general, attempt to escape from it however, over the long haul, this type of shirking, for the most part, doesn't function admirably.

Staying away appears not working in light of the fact that enthusiastic torment is a piece of life. Just we can't maintain a strategic distance from it. Everybody has agonizing sentiments sooner or later, for example, trouble, tension or outrage.

The contrast between overcoming the agony or propping it up and exacerbating it can be the means by which we decide to react to difficult emotions.

Truly, attempting to maintain a strategic distance from or forestall upsetting contemplations and sentiments could be what adds to mental clutters and wretchedness. Of model, an individual who has experienced a horrendous accident might be consistently overwhelmed by injury recollections just as dread and nervousness.

As a result, the individual can attempt to acquire transitory alleviation by medications or liquor (self-sedating), which may help in the short run, however, over the long haul, the liquor or medications will do nothing to calm the agony. At that point, the enduring is relied upon to deteriorate — and put in a large group of different issues.

What Could Be Done?

ACT is a restorative methodology dependent on the thought that misery isn't actuated by encountering enthusiastic agony yet by our endeavors to evade the torment. ACT is utilized for the determination of depression and other dysfunctional behaviors.

ACT's definitive objective is to help individuals both be open and ready to investigate their internal emotions by centering consideration, making an effort not to get away or maintain a strategic distance from torment (since that is inconceivable), yet carry on with significant life.

Here are the 5 Acceptance and Commitment Therapy (ACT) Goals for PTSD and numerous other well-being issue: If you decide to have this treatment and seek after these objectives, this is what you can hope to learn and accomplish:

Perceiving: That Trying to Escape Emotional Pain Never Will Work

ACT Therapists call this objective imaginative misery.It's reached when you see that all the stuff you've managed to do to stop emotional pain doesn't work, and there'll definitely never be a successful way to remove emotional pain from your life altogether.

Learning That Regulation Is the Issue

ACT's second goal is learning that your issues do not arise from the emotional pain itself but from your attempts to control or stop it. In reality, with ACT for PTSD, you might discover that trying to control emotional pain has the opposite effect: Past conceivably making the torment more grounded, you can contribute such a ton of vitality and effort endeavoring to keep up a key good ways from it that you don't have anything left in your life to do positive things.

Believing yourself to be segregated from your insights

Our thoughts are dependable. An individual who has encountered a horrible mishap may have musings of being a terrible individual or of being "broken" or "harmed," yet however these considerations may feel genuine, they are just contemplations. They're not so much a portrayal of what is reality.

A third objective in ACT for PTSD is for individuals to gain from their contemplations to "make a stride back" and not get tied up with them as truth. An advantage is only an inclination. It is anything but an impression of who the individual truly is.

Stopping the battle

At this phase during your PTSD ACT, you'll be urged to stop your back-and-forth with your emotions and musings. The point is to relinquish endeavors to stay away from or control your musings and emotions and rather work on being both open and ready to encounter considerations and affections for what they are and not what you think they are (for instance, awful or risky).

Resolving to Action

For individuals with PTSD, maintaining a strategic distance from enthusiastic torment requires a gigantic measure of vitality. It can gobble your life up. As a result, you may not place a lot of time or vitality into carrying on with a significant and remunerating life. Henceforth, a definitive objective of your ACT for PTSD is to distinguish regions of significance in your life (alluded to as "values" in ACT) and to build the time you spend doing things that are predictable with those qualities, paying little heed to what feelings or considerations may emerge.

For instance, an individual who has experienced rape, while esteeming closeness and commonality, may stay away from or feel on edge about getting into connections once more.

In ACT, individuals are urged to take part in activities that are predictable with their qualities (for example, reconnecting with an old companion) while being open and ready to feel any nervousness that may result.

Not keeping away from that tension keeps it from deteriorating, and it is less inclined to meddle with the quest for an important life by the individual.

Picking ACT treatment for your PTSD

Numerous advisors presently have some expertise in ACT treatment, yet different techniques are additionally accessible to seek after this treatment. There are numerous manners by which individuals with PTSD can seek after acknowledgment and duty treatment, from essential consideration facilities to day-long gathering workshops, to cell phone applications, to telehealth choices.

TREATMENT OF ANXIETY WITH ACT

Acknowledgment and responsibility Therapy (ACT) for nervousness issue is an inventive acknowledgment put together to conduct treatment in concentrations with respect to lessening the social administrative capacity of tension and related insights and has a solid spotlight on social change steady with customer esteems. Along these lines, this remedial strategy has two primary objectives: (a) preparation acknowledgment of issue stricken unhelpful contemplations and emotions that cannot and should not have to be controlled, and (b) duty and activity to carry on with an actual existence through chosen esteem. This shows why ACT is about acknowledgment and simultaneously, it's about change. Applied to uneasiness issue, individuals figure out how to stop the fight with their misery related torment and assume responsibility for it by making a move that pushes them toward their ideal life objectives (values). This technique likewise instructs patients' abilities to acknowledge and watch troublesome musings and emotions similarly as they are to change or decline undesirable considerations and sentiments as opposed to educating "progressively, extraordinary, better" systems to. In this manner, staying away from tension alongside adaptability because of it and different types of passionate distress gives a circumstance to people who follow up on them toward their picked life objectives in any event, when there are upsetting considerations, emotions, and body sensations.

ACT alluded to uneasiness issues as well as tried to limit extraordinary nervousness pain and screen pointless private occasions alongside down-directing experiential shirking endeavors.

Right now, meetings of ACT were treated with three back to back referrals looking for treatment for uneasiness issue at a private practice.

The aftereffects of this investigation demonstrated three back to back cases that exhibited uneasiness issues were treated for nervousness issue convention with ten meetings of a comparable ACT. Members show pretreatment clinically noteworthy and post-treatment enhancements in the recurrence of uneasiness issue. This arrangement of cases has both clinical and test suggestions. This is the main investigation we know about tentatively utilizing ACT for uneasiness issue to follow changes in tension and evasion utilizing a period arrangement structure. Information from three cases isn't complete in any capacity, yet the consistency is outstanding over each of the three members. These discoveries bolster a procedure of progress, including modification of the nervousness work over its seriousness. This information proposes that a tension issue can be dealt with effectively by concentrating on the uneasiness' useful effect on conduct over nervousness level.

In assessing the exact status of ACT, disregard that one of the essential expectations of its creators was to make a comprehensively pertinent trans-symptomatic model, including the treatment of issues that don't fit flawlessly into analytic classes.The content of ACT protocols varies little between applications, and this creates potential efficiencies in training and skill development in settings where it is difficult to restrict the range of complaints presented. To date, no systematic investigation has been carried out into ACT's potential cost-effectiveness. There is some indication from Luoma and his colleague that ACT is related to accessing more therapy, which can be advantageous if the alternative reduces the cost of treatment and also develops greater independence and self-management skills of clients compared to alternative therapy. Such possibilities require more study.

Ipso facto, ACT helped the patient introduce the sense that fighting and control can actually interfere with the patient's day-to-day functioning and life-aim achievement, and then briefly explore that notion in terms of the life experiences of patients. Recognizing and then removing approaches that have not helped people improve their lives are directed at maintaining the quality of life and have not actually provided any meaningful relief from pain. This method was a constructive approach to customer behavioral change with an emphasis on improving quality of life. That's why the ACT program's perhaps most necessary aim is to encourage patients to go in the direction of life-aim. The accentuation was on indicating patients' affirmation and care capacities as strategies for making sense of how to totally and for what they are seeing bothersome apprehension related responses (for instance, thinking as thoughts, physical sensations as physical sensations, pictures as pictures, notions as feelings). The point was to figure out how to remain on edge.This phase is described as "getting ready to face fear with careful acknowledgement so you can get on with your life" Practice participation offered a major incentive for patients to build and cope with the ability to encounter depression and GAD.

Acceptance and Commitment Group Therapy for Health Anxiety

Previously, it was named hypochondriasis and now medical anxiety disorder in DSM-5, causes distress and higher health care costs. In 126 patients with severe health anxiety and without psychosis or bipolar disorder (mean age, 36; 71 % female), researchers in Scandinavia conducted a randomized, waitlist-controlled group acceptance and commitment therapy (ACT-G) preliminary for well-being uneasiness. ACT utilizes methodologies of acknowledgment, care, and conduct change to assist patients with tolerating frightful and maintained a strategic distance from contemplations, sentiments, and recollections. It explains individual qualities and focuses on and seeksout change in conduct.

The waitlist treatment required routine services and a report of general management advice to the primary care provider. ACT-G, conveyed in gatherings of nine patients each and two specialists for every gathering, included nine 3-hour week by week meetings over multiple months and later a promoter meeting (all out treatment, 30 hours).

The ACT-G group showed significantly greater progress in sickness anxiety than the waitlist community (the main outcome; 22 points on a 100-point scale vs. no change), total pronounced increase levels (48% vs. 16%), and quality of life, and emotional distress mitigation. The treatment was very satisfied with more than 80 % of ACT-G patients. Be that as it may, during the mediation or at half-year development, the gatherings didn't contrast in help-chasing for ailment concerns.

ACT FOR STRESS RELIEF

We cannot generally change the conditions that cause us stress, and some of the time, we cannot impact them. When resources are low, you can't always quit a difficult job or get a bonus, and there will always be those hard people you just need to work with.

Some pressure should be overseen, and when you discover methodologies that assist you with managing worry such that limits its negative impacts, it tends to be groundbreaking.
One of these techniques isacceptanceand commitment therapy (ACT), which is becoming more common. This is a method of counseling related to cognitive-behavioral therapy, which many trials have shown to be beneficial in managing stress. ACT incorporates the use of stressor tolerance in one's life and relaxation techniques combined in various ways with commitment and behavior-changing approaches that may improve psychological and emotional resilience.

ACT History

This methodology was initially called "complete separating," and was established by therapist Steven C. Hayes in 1982. From that point forward, it has been fleshed out and progressed in the direction of a progressively powerful way to deal with change. There are now many specific ACT guidelines that vary depending on the situation and level of tension encountered and the environment. For example, there is a brief version of ACT, also known as FACT, called "focused acceptance and commitment therapy."

The point of ACT (and FACT) isn't to expel troublesome sentiments yet to be OK with them and grasp them, in this way making more noteworthy closeness with them so individuals can move past the obstructions such emotions construct. Acceptance and commitment counseling encourage people to open themselves up to uncomfortable emotions and to try not to overreact to them or to avoid situations in which they are called upon. Its therapeutic effect is a positive emotional "upward spiral," where better feeling leads to a better understanding of the truth.

The ACT principles commonly use six core principles to assist clients in developing psychological flexibility.

Cognitive defusion: techniques of learning to of the propensity towards reifying feelings, pictures, emotions, and memories.

Acceptation: Allowing emotions to come and go without having to fight for them.

Connect with the present moment: Here and now consciousness, felt with transparency, curiosity, and receptivity.

The self-observing: Accessing a transcendent sense of self, an unchanging continuity of consciousness.

Values: To find what makes a difference most to oneself.

Submitted activity: Setting and completing goals dependably as per values.

Correlational proof has discovered that numerous types of psychopathology are anticipated by the absence of mental adaptability. A 2005 meta-examination demonstrated that, contingent upon the measure, the six ACT standards speak to 16 to 29 percent of the benchmark fluctuation in psychopathology (general emotional well-being, gloom, nervousness) utilizing correlation techniques.

ACT-Based Strategies:

Mindfulness and Meditation

Because the main goal of ACT is to accept one's present circumstances, become more comfortable with them, and then be empowered to move beyond them with minimal stress, meditation is an extremely useful tool for this kind of stress.

The practice of mindfulness and meditation can enable you to practice the awareness of stressors and then let go of the need to respond. This can limit the pressure that you feel just as the inclination that a considerable lot of us face when we feel caught to overcompensate to the pressure we experience. This can come as ruminations, ruinous perspectives, and different pressure worsening examples that a significant number of us enjoy whether we know it.

Many meditation techniques that can be used to relieve stress are as follows.

Re-evaluation

We cannot always change what we are experiencing, but we can change the way we think about these experiences. That is ACT's core belief.

Changing your thoughts about the stress you experience can come in the form of cognitive restructuring or cognitive re-evaluations, where you work actively to select new ways of viewing the same situation. These views may not be the first thoughts you had on the subject, but they can be aligned with the realities of the situation just as much.

For example, when facing a challenge that feels beyond your capabilities (a commonly stressful situation), "I'm failing in this," it can be changed to, "I'm having a difficult time with this. It's all part of the process, though, and I'll eventually get it." Similarly, "This shouldn't happen to me," it can be changed to, "We're all facing challenges, and here's one of mine. We can feel overpowered by a for all intents and purposes incomprehensible errand when we believe we have to battle against something that may not really be alterable. At the point when we acknowledge a circumstance and let go of our own need to control it (which is frequently unthinkable, in any case), this can want to lift a load off our shoulders and can extraordinarily soothe the pressure of whatever circumstance we face.

"Taking companions" with the circumstances we had been battling with can be a freeing procedure and, curiously, can assist us with moving from feeling "stuck" and "caught" into a spot where we perceive "what is" and what should be possible about it.

Choosing Purposeful Action

A primary objective of ACT is to choose an action that can be done to step in a constructive, productive direction. One approach that can assist with this is to maximize the positive experiences you get so you can build an "upward curve of positivity." Another is to actually look at the situation you are in (and acknowledge that condition) and then search choices you can choose from within this scenario rather than trying to change the fact itself by struggling against the overall circumstances.

This can be accomplished with the help of a therapist, a journaling practice, or talks with an understanding friend.

In the end, strategies based on ACT can be liberating and empowering. Acknowledgment of life's difficulties and pushing ahead can fabricate trust and inward quality and can assist you with moving past critical measures of pressure. Practice can make impeccable with this methodology.

CHAPTER 6

ACT TRAINING
THE BEST WAY TO PICK THE RIGHT GUIDE FOR YOU ATC TRAINGING

A Handy Guide to Our ACT Learning/training Series

You are a mental health professional who has had some contact with acceptance and commitment therapy (ACT), whether you are an accomplished ACT therapist or just read of ACT, and you want to know how to get going. You might have read ACT books and have a craving for hands-on training. And, how do you realize what ACT preparation is appropriate for you?

The good news is, for every level of clinical experience, this part of the book covers ACT training. And luckily for all the Acceptance and Commitment Therapy Training Series, you have this handy guide! This ACT series brings together professionals who have only heard of ACT to fluidly implement it with clients on a daily basis.

ACT BootCamp: Introduction to Implementation

For professionals with little to no prior experience with ACT and those who wish to deepen their ACT practice. Learn the foundations of the psychological flexibility model, and develop an initial set of skills in ACT. Comprehend the basics of social edge hypothesis—the language hypothesis and the comprehension on which ACT is constructed. It's obvious, do, get their criticism. Perceiving mental rigidity in customers continuously, get hands-on, guided practice, and figure out how to react smoothly from all focuses on the hexaflex. Investigate how ACT revives your treatment relationship with customers. Close with one day of a viable survey of what you've realized, fortifying the devices and procedures to work with clients. To get your inquiries replied and manufacture network, go to night meetings for all-out inundation into ACT.

Consider going to an ACT BootCamp on the off chance that you: are keen on ACT and are prepared to make a plunge Are rehearsing ACT however don't have numerous partners who can ricochet thoughts off Are rehearsing ACT and need to improve your training, submersion style.

ACT II: Introduction to ACT For experts with practically zero past involvement in ACT

Get familiar with the establishments of the mental adaptability model, and de Say, say, get their surveys.

Plunge into the hypothesis of social edges—the language hypothesis and the comprehension whereupon ACT is based. Get familiar with the hexaflex (adaptable contact with the present minute, intellectual defusion, acknowledgment, self-as-setting, values, submitted activity) and fundamental ACT forms while adding ACT similitudes and methods to your restorative tool stash. At an ACT I, you will leave the six fundamental procedures of ACT's Psychological Flexibility Model with an experiential comprehension, just as how to apply it to case conceptualization and treatment arranging. You will increase pragmatic abilities to meet customers where they are, and cultivate their eagerness to change and receptiveness.

Think about going to an ACT I on the off chance that you: are keen on ACT and need to begin utilizing it with clients. Want to comprehend the Psychological Flexibility Model and how incredible the six procedures of ACT can be with your most troublesome clients. Need some new apparatuses to support your ACT II remedial tool compartment: Clinical abilities.Experts who practice ACT, however, need increasingly functional experience. As you manufacture a strong premise in the dynamic utilization of ACT intercessions, you will see, do and get input. This workshop is specifically intended for people who are reasonably familiar with mid-level ACT terms, especially the six core ACT processes (meaningfulness, self-as-context, acceptance, defusion, values, and commitment). If you're already studying the pattern in your practice, or if you've undergone a beginning ACT class, you can be sure that you'll profit from ACT II. Because frankly, even professional ACT practitioners can consider plenty of new learning experiences that will improve their skills and make them more efficient.

The goal is to be able to use evidence-based systems that are related to evidence-based practices that address issues and foster human development. This is a type of evidence-based treatment that is quite distinct from the "syndrome guidelines" schemes of the age we finally put in the rearview mirror.

The outcome? A superior comprehension of the model and the capacity to perceive and react progressively to customers ' rigidity. Net result: Better clinical results.Read more on our ACT II workouts!

Consider attending an ACT II if you:
- Are practicing ACT and it's going well, but you want more hands-on practice
- Are practicing ACT but find yourself stumbling from process to process in session
- Are practicing ACT and feeling rigid or "by the book "–you're struggling to embody the practice
- Feel stuck with ACT and aren't sure how to unstick

ACT III: Mastering ACT

This is meant for professionals actively using ACT who intend to make use of it in their most complex cases. It is a master class that is all about the art and science of doing ACT well with all of your clients—mostly for those you only meet for limited sessions.

Train your hardest cases and work with master ACT trainers to solve your biggest challenges. Develop inside the therapy room an understanding of the intra-and interpersonal processes that occur. Foster a deeper understanding of how both you and your customers impact your own behaviors. Get escalated practice at the time to direct useful examination, and afterward apply ACT answers for your discoveries.

Think about going to an ACT III on the off chance that you:

•	Have been rehearsing ACT normally and need assistance applying it to your mind-boggling cases

•	Want to fortify the helpful relationship with your customers

•	Want to bring a profound plunge into your own practices inside your training Want to expand your ease when rehearsing ACT

Acknowledgment and Commitment Therapy (ACT) urges individuals to grasp their contemplations and emotions.

From the outset, it might appear to be confounding, however, ACT combined with care based treatment offers clinically successful treatment. All things considered: fleeing from any issue just expands the arrangement's separation. The least demanding approach to escape is to take care of the issue.

ACT and Mindfulness-Based Cognitive Therapy (MBCT) would all be able to profit by ailments, for example, dread, sorrow, Ptsd, addictions, and substance misuse.

ACT creates mental adaptability and is a type of conduct treatment that joins the abilities of care with self-acknowledgment practice. Duty assumes a key job in planning to be all the more tolerating of your considerations and sentiments. On account of ACT, rather than overlooking the stresses, you vow to handle the issue head-on. Picture adding to acts that will assist you in facilitating your experience and take on any undertaking.

ACT is compelling for a wide scope of mental issue and it additionally goes about as an invigorating and moving self-assurance point of view.

Acknowledgment is an option in contrast to our impulse to abstain from contemplating encounters that are negative-or possibly negative. It is the dynamic decision to acknowledge the nearness of upsetting encounters, without attempting to deny or change them.

Acknowledgment isn't an ACT objective; however, it is an apparatus to advance change that will prompt positive results.

Psychological Defusion alludes to procedures intended to change how an individual responds to their considerations and sensations. Acknowledgment and Commitment Therapy doesn't expect to confine our entrance to negative encounters, but instead to address them and turn out then again with a decreased spotlight on them.

Present Being can be comprehended as the act of being aware of the present minute, without making a decision about the experience. That is, it implies recognizing what's happening without attempting to anticipate or change the experience.

Self as context is the possibility that an individual isn't just the aggregate of their feelings, considerations, or encounters. The procedure of "self as setting" offers the elective idea that outside of the present understanding, there is self.

We are not exactly what is befalling us. We are the ones who have encountered what is befalling us.

Right now, are the characteristics that we decide to progress in the direction of at some random minute. We as a whole hold esteem which manage our activities, deliberately or unknowingly. In ACT, we use apparatuses to assist us with living our lives as indicated by the qualities we hold dear.

At last, ACT expects to assist individuals with adding to practices that will assist them with accomplishing their long haul objectives and carry on with a real existence good with their convictions. Increments of positive conduct cannot emerge without being aware of how we are affected by a particular conduct.

ACT isn't so unmistakable from other helpful treatments; it just anxieties resilience instead of dismissal, and in this manner differs from numerous different types of treatment. This disparity from most traditional treatment might be followed back to the historical backdrop of Stephen C. Hayes, the executive of ACT.

Steven C. Hayes and Steven C. Hayes, a University of Nevada educator of brain science, created ACT in 1986. His work started with how our inward encounters were impacted by language and thought and established the framework for ACT.

Hayes couldn't help contradicting the need to stay away from and cushion up anguish and torment at whatever point conceivable. He considered agony to be an inalienable and vital piece of human life, just as a wellspring of fulfillment when we are not running from what alarms us.

Steven Hayes is putting forth a convincing defense for acknowledgment and self-sympathy dependent on his own agonizing encounters. His TED Talk on Psychological Flexibility clarifies the preparation for his ACT mental research.

The job of ACT in Psychology and Mindfulness

Acknowledgment and Commitment Therapy depends on the Theory of Relational Frame, a hypothesis dependent on the possibility that the human capacity to relate is the premise of language and cognizance.

Relating incorporates observing the estimations the relationship exists close by.We might be partner an apple with an orange, for instance, yet our capacity to relate permits us to get that despite the fact that they have a comparative shape (round) and work (to be eaten), they have various hues and surfaces.

Rather than most different creatures, the job of ACT in brain research and care apple orange people has an uncanny capacity to relate even unbiased occasions, just as apparently inconsequential words and thoughts.

While this is an invaluable capacity, it additionally encourages negative considerations and self-judgment. On the off chance that we can relate "treat" to the treat eating experience, at that point, we can likewise relate "useless" to feeling we're useless.

Our capacity to shape relationship systems (e.g., I partner the words "orange," "apple," and "pear" to the idea of "organic product") can be a dangerous capacity when nervousness and discouragement influence us.

For example, we may relate "useless" to a capacity to play out my activity and relate "useless" to my life by augmentation. ACT depends on the Theory of Relational Frames.

We regularly make relationship arrangements that are not complimentary or nurturing, yet we can likewise change those connections in the event that we apply attention to acknowledge our emotions and change how we respond and identify with them, rather than endeavoring to keep up a vital good ways from them.

Important things to note about ATC training.

Are you prepared to use ACT as a way of improving your life or your customers? If so, read on to apply the science of acceptance and commitment therapy to your job for excellent resources.

A considerable lot of these are made accessible by the ACT Mindfully association, which is an incredible asset.
Here is a rundown of interesting points right now:

- Consider on the off chance that you need assistance or backing, and who can furnish you with the assistance or bolster you need.
- Talk of whether you've encountered anything specific before, and how you then reacted.
- Consider ways, even in the smallest way, to improve the situation, whether it is in the next few minutes or the next few days.

• If you can't improve your circumstance, be happy to rehearse acknowledgment, and focus on investing your time and vitality in a productive way.

• Ask yourself what the most ideal approach to deal with this situation is, or, as the model goes, how to play the game with the cards you were managing.

• Remember to rehearse self-sympathy; envision a companion or adored one experiencing your experience at the present time, in the event that you need motivation, and reveal to yourself whatever you envision letting them know.

Mental Inflexibility

The degree to which anybody experiences difficulty rehearsing the six center procedures is called mental resoluteness or psychological inflexibility.
The questions chart the reverse of the six central mechanisms as follows:

- The superiority of the conceptualized past or future; minimal self-knowledge (vs. acceptance)
- Fusion (vs. defusion)
- Experiential detachment (vs. being present)
- Attachment to the conceptualized self (vs. self as context)
- Loss of beliefs Clarity / contact (vs. values)
- Unworkable behavior (vs. dedicated intervention)

This arrangement of inquiries is a basic advance towards grasping their encounters and acting to the most profound qualities they hold.

CHAPTER 7

Valuable ACT EXERCISES

This is a snappy exercise for psychological well-being experts to enable their customers to see how counterproductive evasion can be. You will finish up this activity in the accompanying advances: Bring your client a piece of paper and a pen and approach them in the event that they are prepared for composed guidelines.Before the consumer may compose something, pose an obstruction that obstructs the capacity of the customer to see the paper and pen (e.g., a sheet of cardboard, a mask with a severely limited vision, etc.) Ask the customer if they are disturbed by this and if they would rather see how they type. Inform them that the barrier would stay, but they should still try to work around the obstacle in order to write the sentence. Let them fail for 20-30 seconds to see around the obstacle. At this stage, they probably won't have written something understandable Tell the customer about their experience (i.e., "How was it? Was it difficult? Are you able to write the sentence? Could we understand it?") Propose that the customer stop trying to see around the barrier but just agree that it is there and write the sentence anyway.

APPLYING MINDFULNESS TO YOUR THERAPEUTIC PRACTICE

There is a huge difference in the sentence they write when focusing on writing (instead of avoiding); this could probably be more readable. Please point that out to them and help them link between preventing the physical barrier and avoiding emotional pain, and the negative consequences of each.

This exercise can be done on your own or guided by a therapist. Taking these measures will allow you or your customer to realize that pain is an inevitable part of life; if we remove misery, we can reduce happiness as well.

Follow these means to attempt this activity:

Locate an important movement or relationship that you have pulled back from as of late;

Take out a file card or a bit of paper. From one viewpoint, record what you esteem about that action or relationship or what you plan to achieve or become through it;

then again, record the hard considerations and sentiments that occasionally transpire when you make a move to pick up the worth or accomplishments composed on the opposite side;

Put the card in your pocket, wallet, or sack.

Take it out throughout the following week, take a gander at the two sides, and ask yourself whether you're willing to have that card, with both great and awful.

It is possible that you can keep away from the worth and the agony or you can grasp both.

What CarolVivyan says about Exposure to Emotions?

This is a procedure of mindfulness that can defuse a substantial, negative feeling. Follow the means to recharge your emphasis on tolerating your qualities and making a positive move: sit easily in a calm zone. Carry your consideration regarding your body, experience the breathing sentiments without endeavoring to control the breath; note the feeling (s) that you sense, and what it seems like; call the feeling. Perceive what it is and what word best portrays how you feel; recognize feeling as a trademark and normal response to conditions.Don't tolerate or judge it, just let it move through you; investigate the emotion by asking questions such as: How intensely do I feel this emotion? Did my respiration change? What are the sensations which accompany my body? What is my posture like? Do I experience heightened muscle tension? What is my current facial expression? How does that look on my face?
Note the subsequent emotions or conclusions but let them move. When you find yourself concentrating on

any of them, gently bring back your mindto re-centering your breathing, then explore the feeling again. This technique could yield the best results when you start small and work your way up to more intense emotions.

This technique is an extraordinary initial step to begin rehearsing ACT procedures for anybody attempting to. Qualities are an essential bit of acknowledgment and responsibility treatment, as referenced before.

The worksheet Valued Directions provides ten interest areas for the student to consider which are listed below:

- Work/career;
- Intimate relationships;
- Parenting;
- Education/learning/personal growth;
- Friends/social life;
- Health/physical self-care;
- Family of birthplace (or connections other than marriage or child-rearing)
- Spirituality Community life/condition/nature;
- Recreation

The activity at that point requests that the peruser rate the significance of each worth area to two (significant) on a size of zero(not at all significant).

There's nothing wrong with more value of certain fields than others.

In each field, readers then score their satisfaction with their lives on a scale from zero (not satisfied at all) to two (very satisfied).

When the appraisals have been finished, the activity requests that perusers survey any an incentive on the size of essentialness evaluated as one or two and to compose their aims for years to come around there.In other words, write down what you want to achieve, retain, or become in every important area of value.

These are not targets that can be achieved and "checked off," but rather aspirations that are actionable and suit the way you want to conduct your daily life.

This exercise can help explain what is important in your life, what needs to be prioritized. It's better if you have a doctor or a trained specialist to share with them the outcomes and expectations that can be actioned. Whether you are actually undergoing counseling or not, it is still a successful practice.

Metaphors also play an important role in acceptance and commitment therapy. They give customers a straightforward method for seeing how their sentiments and musings impact their activities, permitting individuals to perceive how our practices are influenced by changing our considerations.

Here are three of our preferred significant analogies for ACT.

The Metaphor Sailing Boat

This analogy utilizes the setting of a little cruising pontoon with "you" as a mariner. At times waves send water over the surface and into the boats, permitting wet feet to disturb you. The pontoon has a bailer to spare the water, so you figure out how to utilize that gas.

So one day, you begin bailing when an especially enormous wave breaks over the side and leaves water in your pontoon. You may continue The Sailing Boat Metaphor acting to bail gently or attentively, but you may eventually find yourself bailing frantically or violently to get out of all this water.

Have you noticed what happens to your boat while you were bailing? Where are they headed? Where did it drift to? Would it be fair to say that you bailed up more than just sailing?

Then imagine taking a look at the bailer and seeing it's just a sieve, full of holes? Which is it you would do?

The implicit purpose of bailing water here is likely to get your boat back on track— once you get rid of the water boat. But if your device doesn't suit the mission, you'll find yourself trying to get out of any water, let alone steer your ships.

The question is, would you rather be on a boat that only has a little water in the bottom but is drifting without direction, or on a boat that may have quite a bit of water in the bottom but heads in the direction you want to go?

This representation can support you or your clients acknowledge two things: The methods we use to manage our upset musings and emotions are instruments like the bailer and the sifter, and some are superior to other people.At times working frantically to stay away from wet feet (or other difficult or awkward sentiments) makes us so off course; the "wet feet" interruption and battle turns into our squares to accomplish our objectives, not the waves.

The Mind Bully Metaphor
This metaphor is intended for people who have a particular emotion or illness, such as frustration, fear, or depression.

The mind bully is our particular problem in this metaphor: it is an incredibly large and powerful bully.

We are pulling to and fro on a rope on inverse sides of a pit as the Mind Bully attempts to make us fall into the pit.

At the point when we pull on the rope, tune in and focus on the beast or even trust it, we are really taking care of it.Like any bully, as we interact with it, the Mind Bully can only hurt us and believe the negative things it tells. To put it another way, do not let your mind bully your body.

What do you think would happen if we dropped it, instead of pulling on the rope? The Mind Bully might still be there, hurling its insults and meanness, but it couldn't pull us to the pit anymore.

The less we feed the Mind Bully, the littler it will get, and the calmer it will. Maybe, in the long run, we will even develop compassion for this miserable animal and miracle why it says mean considerations like that. By seeing and recognizing it, we quit taking care of the Mind Bully, however moving our consideration away from it as opposed to accepting what it says. Focusing on a quick practice in mindfulness can be an extraordinary method to do this.

The Quicksand Metaphor
Quicksand is a loose, wet sand patch that can't sustain weight like dry sand can. Instead of seeking a solid footing, you start sinking as you walk into quicksand.

Basic information is that battling sand trap just expands the rate and it sucks you down into its profundities. At the point when you put more weight on one foot to attempt to lift the other, you simply sink into the pit further. The lower you fall, the more you endure. Wonderment! Wonder!

The solution to surviving quicksand is to spread your body weight and move slowly over a large surface area.

Rather than attempting to fight the sand trap, disregard your battling impulses and rather rests on your back.

It is nonsensical, however the less you battle, and the simpler it is to get away, the more you acknowledge your present circumstance and grasp weakness.

A similar rule applies to agony, enduring, and realizing when to request help. The more we fight and fight against it, the more we drag ourselves down deeper rather than accepting our situation.

When we agree that the pain is imminent, we are more likely to survive and come out faster and more effectively from the other side.

ACT FOR TREATING DISORDERS

Unlike mindfulness practice, ACT can be used in the life of any person, dealing with general anxiety symptoms, chronic pain, insomnia, OCD, eating disorders, and social anxiety.

General and Social Anxiety Disorders

Numerous examinations show the constructive outcomes this type of treatment has on patients with tension battles.
For example, one study showed that college students receiving ACT treatment enjoyed less stress with regard to academic concerns, decreased symptoms of anxiety and depression, increased overall mental health, and increased considerate acceptance (Levin, Haeger, Pierce, &Twohig, 2017).

Another study reiterated these positive anxiety impacts and showed that ACT delivered over the internet could be as effective as ACT delivered by a therapist (Ivanova et al., 2016).

The members right now show a decline all in all and social uneasiness, regardless of whether in the "care as typical" classification or the ACT people group on the web.
In many cases of chronic pain, Chronic Pain Acceptance, and Commitment Therapy has been found to improve quality of life— even without affecting the pain level experienced.

One examination demonstrated that malignancy patients getting ACT treatment detailed noteworthy enhancements in tolerating their conditions and finding expanded significance throughout everyday life, even while experiencing torment (Datta, Aditya, Chakraborty, Das, and Mukhopadhyay, 2016);

Another study also found that ACT improves psychological flexibility and reduces depressive symptoms, even if there is still chronic pain (Scott, Hann, McCracken, 2016).

This result was confirmed by another review, stating that physical and emotional functionality increased with ACT, even with no associated pain reduction (Vowles, Witkiewitz, Levell, Sowden, & Ashworth, 2017).

The same thing is applicable to depression. ACT has been found to support impacts in individuals with misery. One investigation found that ACT decreased the seriousness of burdensome side effects for discouraged veterans and self-destructive musings (Walser, Garvert, Karlin, Trockel, Ryu, and Taylor, 2015).

ACT additionally decreased sorrow and nervousness related mental rigidity and misery in more seasoned grown-ups, even with just a short course from a fledgling ACT specialist (Roberts, 2016).

CHAPTER 8

OBSESSIVE-COMPULSIVE DISORDER (OCD)

ACT CAN ALSO HELP PATIENTS SUFFERING FROM OCD.

An overview of the quantitative research carried out in this area has shown that ACT treatment for OCD is as effective as the "treatment as usual" approach, including cognitive behavioral therapy (Bluett, Homan, Morrison, Levin &Twohig, 2014).

At last, ACT has likewise been effectively applied to patients experiencing dietary problems. A case-arrangement study on ladies with Binge Eating Disorder indicated that the members improved with ACT application (Hill, Masuda, Melcher, Morgan, and Twohig, 2015).

One patient even arrived at a point where her indications never again met the clinical meaning of voraciously consuming food issues, while both demonstrated expanded adaptability in their self-perception.

Toward the finish of the investigation, members who got treatment that included ACT were bound to accomplish positive results in an examination on patients with anorexia (Parling, Cernvall, Ramklint, Holmgren and Ghaderi, 2016).

Applying ACT in Group Therapy

Acknowledgment and Commitment Therapy might be applied at a solitary level, however, it is likewise compelling when conveyed through a treatment gathering. The Association for Contextual Behavioral Science recognizes the efficacy of group ACT therapies for anger, depression and general anxiety, social anxiety, chronic pain, and adolescent struggles.

The Houston Community Psychotherapy Association reiterates the importance of community ACT counseling, emphasizing that a community environment can provide incentives for participants to interact and benefit from each other, gain the support they may urgently need, and cultivate positive vulnerability.

Course Summary ACT is a contextually oriented form of cognitive behavioral psychotherapy that utilizes awareness and behavioral stimulation to improve the interpersonal resilience of a person— his / her ability to engage in values-based, positive behaviors when enduring stressful perceptions, emotions, or feelings. ACT defines this through six main processes: recognition of private experiences; cognitive defusion (i.e., changing the nosy jobs of feelings and other private occasions); staying alert, having a feeling of self-point of view; characterizing values; and taking an interest in conduct.The first four steps describe a cognitive response to ACT, and the last two identify the behavioral reinforcement approach to ACT.

ACT is conveyed to customers in one-on-one meetings, in little gatherings or bigger workshops, or in books or other media, through data introduction, discourse, and the utilization of similitudes, representation activities, and schoolwork practices. Contingent upon the necessities of the customer or treatment supplier, the number, recurrence and length of the meetings and the general span of the intercession can change.

Program Goals
The overall objectives of Acceptance and Commitment Therapy (ACT) are:
- To produce psychological flexibility: the ability to embrace one's thoughts and feelings as they are and to shift attention towards chosen values and actions linked to those values
- Reduce psychopathology
- Increase work performance
- Increase physical health
- Increase quality of life Essential components

The essential components OF ACT were conducted in individual sessions, as well as in small groups with 3-5 members or in large workshops with more than 100 members. There is no recommended definite group

size. The number of participants in a program, amount of sessions, and the actual length of the therapy may vary depending on the client's needs or the care provider's experience.
Because psychological versatility is seen as a central mechanism of behavior, it can be used in many different ways. There is no specific structure of intervention that must be followed. Nonetheless, there are a variety of supportive sources that provide explanations of behaviors and metaphors considered to be successful in affecting relational versatility. Help tools (such as books and videos) should be reviewed so that the clinician can rely on a range of techniques. Clinicians new to ACT are highly recommended to seek some form of oversight or consultation.

Acceptance and Commitment Therapy
ACT varies from CBT in that, instead of questioning distressing feelings by searching for evidence and seeking a more rational response (CBT), in ACT, the feeling is recognized as a concept, e.g., "I'm afraid this boat is going to sink," and then defused using a variety of techniques that may include relaxation, symbols, and vocabulary.

ACT employs three broad categories of methods: conscientiousness, including being present at the moment and strategies of defusion; acceptance; and commitment to acting on principles.

Mindfulness
Mindfulness is a way to observe our experience, without judgment, in the present moment. Mindfulness helps us to' defuse'-away from unhelpful thoughts, reactions, and sensations.

Acceptance
ACT is based on the idea that it only enhances and transforms it into something painful, simply trying to rid oneself of pain and distress. The alternative is to accept it - but that doesn't mean giving up, defeating, or agreeing to suffer. Acceptance is a recognition of and willingness to allow for these experiences.

We learn to make space for painful feelings, ideas, and experiencesto encourage them to be there, to come and to go without us resisting them.

Commitment and Values-based Life
You will strive to liberate yourself from life's constraints and obstacles and see what your life truly needs to be.

Values
Meaning is the course of existence, an inner compass that leads us through all life. Values are different from goal goals. Words often last forever. Perhaps our

headstone dedication is what we would like to be known for, or published as our epitaph.

Values do give meaning and purpose to life.

To order to identify our beliefs, we should talk about what is really essential to us in life, what brings meaning and purpose to our lives.

Is it our partnerships, for example, being a good parent? Is that our jobs, communicating with nature, healthy living, service to the community, or making a difference? Consider what heritage you wish to pass on.

After identifying our values, we know where we want to go in life, in which direction we want to move forward. We could be setting goals along the way.

Knowing our values will help us decide how to respond to stress and hardship. We can still move in the direction and service of our values, despite the way we feel.

The Quicksand

Suppose you find someone standing in the middle of a swimming pool of quicksand-no ropes or tree branches are available. The only way you can improve is through communication with them. The person yells, "HELP! GET ME OUT!" and begins doing what people do-struggling to get out. The effective action to take is to walk, run, step, hop, or jump out of trouble 99.9 % of the time.

Not in quicksand. Typically you need to raise one foot and push the other forward to get out of something. That is a bad idea with quicksand. When one foot is raised, the weight of the entire person lies on the other foot only (half of the former surface area), and the downward pressure doubles. The guy sinks deeper.

As you watch, you see them sinking deeper. Unless you realize how quickly sand operates, you may be yelling at them to lie flat, spread-eagled, optimizing surface communication. Therefore, the person probably won't sink and could roll to safety.

Since the individual is attempting to escape the sand trap, to expand body contact with it, it conflicts with all their common senses. Somebody who battles to escape the mud may never understand that getting with the mud is the savvy and more secure activity.
That can be much like our own lives. The standard problem-solving strategies we employ (sometimes repeatedly for years) to try to deal with the problems we encounter, may be part of the problem itself, just like someone struggling to get out of the quicksand.

ACT promises something very special to help us get out of the quicksand in which we find ourselves but to get along with it. By doing so, we can alleviate our suffering and empower ourselves to lead valued, meaningful, dignified human lives.

ACT is a mental mediation approach characterized by some hypothetical procedures and not a particular innovation. In hypothetical and procedure terms, we can characterize ACT as a mental intercession dependent on present day conduct brain research, including Relational Framework Theory (RFT), which applies procedures of mindfulness and acknowledgment, and procedures of responsibility and change of conduct to make mental adaptability.

ACT's central idea is that psychological trauma is usually caused by the interaction of human language and thought, through direct experience regulation over human behavior. It is suggested that psychological inflexibility results through experiential detachment, emotional entanglement, attachment of a conceptualized self, loss of contact with the real and subsequent failure to take appropriate disciplinary action with regards to fundamental beliefs.

Buttressed by RFT, a thorough fundamental research program on a related language and cognizance hypothesis. ACT takes the view that endeavoring to change troublesome contemplations and sentiments as a methods for adapting can be counterproductive, yet there are new, ground-breaking options accessible, including acknowledgment, mindfulness, psychological defusion, values, and submitted activity.

Research appears to show these techniques are gainful to a wide scope of clients. ACT shows customers and advisors the same how to intellectually change the operations of troublesome private encounters as opposed to disposing of them by any stretch of the imagination. That persuasive methodology has been appeared to assist customers with managing a wide scope of wellbeing conditions from sorrow, uneasiness, torment, abuse of medications, and even insane manifestations. The advantages are as significant for the clinician as they are for the customers: exactly, ACT has been appeared to reduce specialist wear out rapidly. We're currently finding that these equivalent components assist us with comprehension and improve various other social issues, including fields, for example, enthusiastic inclination, work execution, or the powerlessness to learn new things.

Pathology model

From the point of view of ACT and RFT, whereas psychological problems may arise from the general absence of relational skills (for example on account of mental impediment), the essential wellspring of psychopathology (just as a procedure that intensifies the effect of different wellsprings of psychopathology) is the manner by which language and cognizance connect with direct possibilities so as to deliver failure. In ACT and RFT, this sort of mental rigidity is contended to rise up out of frail or unhelpful logical command over language forms themselves, and the psychopathology model is in this way connected point-to-point with the fundamental investigation RFT gives. It gives a center level clarification that is open and experimentally significant, associated near increasingly conceptual essential standards.

Subjective combination is a center procedure that can prompt pathology, alluding to the predominance of conduct administrative capacities by social systems, situated specifically on the inability to recognize the procedure and results of social reaction. Human conduct in settings that encourage such combination is guided more by generally unyielding verbal systems than by natural possibilities that are reached. In certain conditions, this is fine, yet in others, it increments unfortunate mental rigidity. As a result, individuals can act in a way that is contradictory with what the world offers that is essential to the qualities and goals picked. The structure or substance of comprehension isn't legitimately alarming from an ACT and RFT perspective, except if logical highlights lead this intellectual substance to direct human activity in an unhelpful way.

The social and verbal culture holds basically the practical structures which seem to have such harmful impacts. There are many. A strict setting treats images (e.g., the idea, "life is sad") as one would call it (i.e., a genuinely miserable life). A setting of reason-giving bases activity or inaction on the built "causes" of one's own conduct too much, particularly when those procedures point to non-manipulable "causes, for example, adapted private occasions. As an essential objective and metric of fruitful living, a setting of experiential control, centers around controlling enthusiastic and psychological states.

Subjective combination bolsters experiential evasion—in any event, while doing so causes social damage, endeavoring to modify the structure, recurrence, or situational affectability of private occasions. The alleged "terrible" sentiments are verbally envisioned, estimated, and opposed in view of the relevant and social associations found in human language. Experiential shirking depends on this common procedure of language—a wonder that the network at that point enhances into a general accentuation on "feeling better" and forestalling distress. Tragically, endeavors to maintain a strategic distance from cumbersome private occasions will in general increment their commonsense significance—both on the grounds that they become progressively normal, and in light of the fact that these avoidance systems are frequently mentally identified with conceptualized negative results—and along these lines will in general limited the scope of exercises that are satisfactory on the grounds that numerous propensities would trigger such feared private occasions.

The popular desire for reason-giving and the functional utility of human symbolic actions pull the individual into efforts even when futile to understand and explain psychological occurrences. Contact with the present minute decreases as people live "in their minds." The conceptualized past and future, and the conceptualized self, acquire administrative control over conduct, contributing further to rigidity. Of example, being correct about who is accountable of personal pain may become more essential than coping more efficiently with the past one has; maintaining a verbal understanding of oneself (e.g., being a survivor, never being upset, becoming abused, etc.) may be more relevant than participating in more workable types of actions that do not suit the verbalisation. In addition, since feelings and considerations are normally utilized as explanations behind different activities, reason-offering will, in general, attract the person to concentrate more on the world inside as the correct wellspring of social guideline, further worsening experiential examples of evasion. The outcome is mental firmness indeed.

In the realm of open conduct, this means that long haul wanted life characteristics — values — assume a lower priority toward increasingly prompt objectives of being correct, looking acceptable, feeling better, protecting a conceptualized self, and so forth. Beyond relief from psychological pain, people lose touch with what they want in life. Patterns of action emerge and are gradually dominating in the repertoire of the person, detached from long-term desired living qualities. Behavioral repertoires are narrow and less sensitive to the current context, as they allow valued actions. Effectiveness service persistence and change is less likely.

The Six Key Processes of ACT

ACT's overall goal is to improve relational flexibility—the capacity to more thoroughly experience the present moment as a conscious human being, and alter or continue in actions when doing so meets desired purposes. Psychological stability is assessed by way of six main ACT mechanisms. Each of these areas is conceptualized as a positive psychological ability, not merely a method of psychopathological avoidance.

Acceptance

Acceptance is given as a remedy to experiential refusal.Acceptance requires the full and conscientious acceptance of those private events that are brought on by one's past without undue attempts to change their frequency or shape, particularly when doing so would cause psychological damage. For example, people with anxiety are encouraged to experience fear as a sensation, completely and without defence; pain patients are offered strategies that allow them to let go of a pain problem, and so on. In ACT, acceptance (and defusion) isn't an end in itself. Instead, acceptance is promoted as a way of increasing value-based action.

Cognitive Defusion

Psychological defusion methods endeavor to adjust the undesirable elements of considerations and other private occasions, as opposed to endeavoring to modify their affectability to frame, recurrence or circumstance.Saying differently, ACT attempts to change the manner in which one communicates with or responds to emotions by establishing ways in which their unhelpful roles decrease.

There are hundreds of such techniques developed for a broad range of clinical presentations. For example, by assigning it a shape, size, colour, intensity, or type, a negative thought could be viewed dispassionately, echoed vigorously until only the sound remains, or regarded as an objectively observable occurrence. A person may praise their minds for such an interesting thought, mark the thinking process ("I'm thinking I'm not good"), or explore the past perceptions, emotions, and memories that arise while they're observing the thought. These techniques seek to reduce the abstract consistency of the meaning, undermining the tendency to treat the idea as what it relates to ("I am not good") rather than what it is actually perceived to be (e.g., the "I am not pleasant" thinking). The consequence of defusion is typically a decrease in the believability of private occasions, or connection to them, as opposed to a quick change in their recurrence.

Being Present

ACT facilitates constant non-judgmental interaction with the experience of social and environmental incidents. The aim is to have customers experience the world more directly so that their behavior is more flexible, and therefore, their actions are more consistent with the values they hold. This is accomplished by enabling workability to exert more control over behavior and by using language more as a tool for recording and describing events, not just for predicting and judging. A feeling of self called "self as procedure" is effectively supported: the defused, non-critical proceeding with depiction of considerations, sentiments, and other private occasions.

Self as Context

Because of social structures, for example, I versus you, presently versus at that point, and here versus there, human language prompts a feeling of self as a locus or viewpoint and gives typical verbal people an extraordinary, profound side. This thought was one of the seeds from which both ACT and RFT developed, and now there is developing proof of its significance for language capacities, for example, compassion, mind hypothesis, self-sense and such.

To put it plainly, the thought is that "I" rises over enormous arrangements of instances of point of view taking connections (which are classified "deictic connections" in RFT), however since this feeling of self is a setting for verbal information, not excessively information's substance, its impediments cannot be intentionally known. Incompletely on the grounds that one can know about one's own progression of encounters without connection to them or an interest in which specific encounters happen: defusion and acknowledgment are hence supported. In ACT, care activities, illustrations, and experiential procedures encourage one's self as setting.

Qualities

Qualities are chosen characteristics of intentional activity that can never be acquired as an object, however, can be momentarily started up. ACT utilizes an assortment of activities to enable a customer to pick life headings in various areas (e.g., family, vocation, otherworldliness) while undermining verbal procedures that could prompt decisions dependent on evasion, social consistency or combination (e.g., "I should esteem X" or "A great individual would esteem Y" or "My mom needs me to esteem Z"). In ACT, acknowledgment, defusion, being available, etc. are not finishes in themselves; rather, they make the way for a real existence that is increasingly essential, predictable with values.

Submitted Action

At last, ACT empowers the advancement of more prominent and more noteworthy examples of powerful activity connected to the qualities picked. Right now, looks particularly like conventional social treatment, and practically any technique for typically reasonable conduct change can be fitted into an ACT convention, including introduction, ability securing, forming strategies, objective setting, and so forth. Not at all like qualities that are continually introduced, however, never accomplished as an article, solid objectives that are predictable qualities can be accomplished, and ACT conventions quite often include work and schoolwork identified with short-, medium-, and long haul objectives to change conduct. Thus, social change endeavors lead to contact with mental hindrances that are tended to by other ACT forms (acknowledgment, defusion, and so forth.).

Taken all in all, every one of these procedures underpins the other, and all the mental adaptability focused on the procedure of completely reaching the present minute as a cognizant person and persevering or changing conduct at the administration of picked esteems.One can split the six processes into two groupings. Processes of conscientiousness and tolerance include recognition, defusion, interaction with the present moment, and self as meaning.

Nonetheless, these four systems provide a workable attentiveness description of actions (see Fletcher & Hayes in the Suggested Reading list, in the press). Processes of the shift in commitment and actions include interaction with the present moment, self as meaning, beliefs, and determined practice. In the two groupings, contact with the present minute and self as setting happens in light of the fact that all mental movement of cognizant individuals includes the now as known.

What is the distinction ACT vs. CBT?

For those progressively educated, self-bailing, inquisitive potential psychotherapy customers out there, I have made a short depiction of the contrasts between two of the most well-known sorts of treatment that clinicians are utilizing nowadays.I'm not expecting most people to know the differences between therapeutic techniques, but surprisingly, I'm finding that more and more people know this stuff and are really interested in how it works. This is a good thing because you ought to learn what kind of evidence-based therapy your doctor gives you anyway! Here I have included a basic description of both CBT and ACT, and how they are related and distinct in the treatment of depression.

Cognitive behavioral therapy (CBT)

CBT is a psychosocial mediation that is the training most generally used to treat mental scatters. CBT centers around creating individual adapting procedures planned for tackling current issues and changing examples of unhelpful perception (for example, contemplations, convictions, and perspectives). The hidden idea driving CBT is that our musings and sentiments are fundamental to our conduct.

CBT is normally present moment and concentrated on helping customers handle a quite certain issue. Individuals figure out how to distinguish and change damaging or upsetting idea designs that affect conduct throughout treatment. Numerous individuals begin recognizing "center convictions" that have, for quite a long time, directed their feelings and practices. CBT causes individuals to see musings which lead to their torment. "I'm continually going to be apathetic, and I'm continually going to be discouraged."

Depiction how CBT functions: A substance state he/she is "miserable things are showing signs of improvement." CBT would enable the person to distinguish the contortion of thought and help them to find considerations, which are sensible and successful in helping them to feel much improved. For example, "I never feel discouraged. At the point when I make a mind-blowing most, there are times. Seeing and changing one's ideas impacts one's very own sentiments.

Further explanation from the example above: When the individual applies a more optimistic (and realistic) thought, their emotion changes (more hopeful) and their behavior changes (going out of bed and walking).

The aim of cognitive behavioral therapy is to show people that while they are unable to control every aspect of the world surrounding them, they will take control of how they perceive and handle things inside their community.

ACT, articulated "act," is a sort of psychotherapy ordinarily portrayed as a type of psychological conduct treatment.It is an empirically based therapeutic technique that utilizes techniques of tolerance, conscientiousness, commitment, and behavior-change to improve psychological versatility.

Instead of trying to teach individuals how to better control their emotions, perceptions, sensations, experiences, and other private events, ACT encourages participants to actually note, accept and embrace their private events, ACT varies from CBT.

ACT is a powerful tool that can reduce suffering without trying to change it by helping one observe thoughts and feelings as they are. ACT also stresses behavior in a manner consistent with valued goals and direction of life.

Example of how ACT works: one would develop depression acceptance and learn to develop a relationship with it instead of avoiding it (what ACT refers to "experiential avoidance"). The fundamental premise of ACT for depression is that while emotional pain hurts, it is the pain process that causes suffering.

ACT has been shown to be effective in treating not only depression but also abuse and anxiety. ACT doesn't attempt to improve or reduce indications but instead plans to enable the individual to quit fixating on their side effects, make new personal conduct standards, and settle on more beneficial decisions. This aides right now to be completely cognizant, and to support or change conduct contingent upon what the circumstance involves.

Looking at ACT and CBT: Defusion versus Restructuring

Some emphasis ondefusion-like procedures has been effectively consolidated in all cases of contemporary modalities of psychotherapy to achieve conduct change. In any case, with regards to psychological social treatment, apparently,defusion and intellectual rebuilding are very chances: the last accept that considerations need to change for conduct to change, while the previous expect that difference in thought is unimportant.

It would suggest at first sight that cognitive behavioral counseling (CBT) is focused on the paradigm in which beliefs trigger problem behaviors and emotions and need to be modified before those behaviors and emotions will improve. Hofman, Asmundson, and Beck took this view and recently stressed that, in cognitive behavioral therapy, "negative emotions and harmful behaviors are the product of dysfunctional thoughts and cognitive distortions." On the off chance that this was a coupling presumption held by all intellectual conduct specialists, it would order the utilization of subjective rebuilding and nullify the utilization of defusion in CBT, since this would be a coupling suspicion held by all psychological conduct advisors.

The utilization of intellectual procedures other than CBT rebuilding is a reasonable game, and contemplations need not cause conduct, however, a potential issue emerges when couple defusion and rebuilding are utilized.

"Defusion basically encourages that musings need not change to change plain conduct, that word wars need not be won before feelings can be acknowledged for what they are. The utilization of rebuilding systems implies that troublesome musings can and should be changed so as to push ahead," says John Blackledge, PhD, specialist and creator of Cognitive Defusion in Practice: A Clinician's Guide to Assess, Observe and Support Change in Your Client.

"Moreover, if an advisor — and by expansion, the customer — isn't unequivocally evident that defusion and rebuilding are only two unique methods for evolving conduct, and that you can act in a way that is conflicting with your considerations, disarray and weakened treatment impacts may result," says Blackledge.

Presently there is no information investigating the impacts of blending defusion and rebuilding strategies—or blending a lessened rendition of the psychological model with the suspicion that musings don't cause conduct—in treatment.

Whenever joined, the most reasonable methodology would presumably include beginning with the express mutual suppositions that: musings once in a while, if at any point, catch the full expansiveness and profundity of the encounters or realities they guarantee to portray. Convincing considerations impact our feelings and practices, yet don't drive us to act or feel in a way steady with them; and defusion and rebuilding. "It may be helpful to change the way you think whenever possible, while at the same time reminding yourself, using defusion strategies, that thoughts need not be changed because they do not capture absolute truth anyway," Blackledge says.

If a provided client gravitates towards methods of transformation and considers them effective in altering many of his feelings, nice. Defusion strategies might be used when restructuring fails, or by clients embracing their message as a frontline approach.

CHAPTER 9

ARE THERE ADVANTAGES OVER TRADITIONAL CBT WITH ACT?

This is an empirical question in the end. Having considered that in a theoretical sense, we can look at the possible advantages.

There are a handful of studies right now that looked directly, and they tend to be medium to small. Only a few are published, and one of those hardly mentions outcome because it was a piece about change process. In this way, we have far to go before this inquiry is exactly replied.

Here are the examinations that have been done as such far: Rob Zettle, who prepared with Beck, did two little randomized preliminaries for wretchedness on ACT versus CT—one utilizing singular ACT and CT, and the other utilizing bunch ACT and CT therapy.Right now, a larger randomized multi-site trial is underway. He found Cohen's d's at post between ACT and CT of 1.23 (individually delivered) and.53 (group) in his two studies (see the ACT Handout), followed by.92 and.75. Yet the N was very small. In the individual study the ACT group was only an N of six and about ten or so in the group study.

The other four studies are brand new and have yet to be published. Ann Branstetter performed a randomized end-stage cancer distress trial. Ann was trained in traditional CBT and used CBT procedures, which she thought would help (such as cognitive restructuring). There was no follow-up because the participants had cancer at the end of the stage, but at week 12 ACT had a Cohen's d of.9 compared to traditional CBT on dying pain. For details, you can email her-she is at the State University of Southwest Missouri.

Jennifer Block's dissertation at Albany (just hired as a faculty member at LaSalle) compared ACT and CBGT in social phobia and found a Cohen's d of.45 in favor of ACT compared to traditional CBT on behavioral (standing up and speaking) measure.

Carmen Luciano's team at Almeria University just did a smoking trial comparing ACT and a CBT package used by a Spanish cancer society and found a Cohen's d of.42 at a one-year smoking cessation follow up.

In a feasibility experiment, RaimoLappalainen and his colleagues at the University of Tampere provide evidence contrasting ACT and standard CBT (using CBT approaches related to behavioral learning, such as skills training or exposure) in a clinic. One ACT and one traditional CBT client were randomly assigned to beginning student therapists (N= 14 each condition). Problems ranged across the usual spectrum of outpatients but were mostly anxiety and depression. On the SCL 90, the post Cohen's d was.62 among ACT and CBT. The outcome got more noteworthy at development. Lappalainen, R., Lehtonen, T., Skarp, E., Taubert, E., Ojanen, M., and Hayes, S. C. (2015). (2007). Effect of models of CBT and ACT utilizing brain research learner specialists: A fundamental controlled preliminary of adequacy. Change of practices, 31, 488-511.There was greater acceptance of ACT participants at phase level; great self-confidence for patients with CBT. Both correlated with results, but only acceptance still relates to results when partial correlations are calculated. Accidentally, the result was not included in the report but in self-confidence, ACT was now significantly better at follow-up than CBT.

At Drexel University, Evan Foreman and James Herbert reported similar data from their clinic: Forman, E. M., Herbert, J. D., Moitra, E., Yeomans, P. D. Geller and P. A. (2015). (2007). A randomized controlled preliminary of acknowledgment and responsibility treatment and psychological treatment for uneasiness and despondency for adequacy. Alteration of conduct, 31(6), 772–799.In this study, 101 heterogeneous outpatients were randomly assigned either to traditional CT or to ACT reporting moderate to severe levels of anxiety or depression. It employed 23 junior therapists. Members getting CT and ACT showed critical and comparable enhancements in gloom, tension, working challenges, personal satisfaction, life fulfillment, and clinician-evaluated working. "Observing" and "describing" one's interactions induced outcomes for those in the CT community compared to those in the ACT category, and for those in the ACT group, "experiential evasion," "acting with sensitivity," and "acceptance" produced performance.

It is also known that ACT methods can empower behavioral methods (which, by the way, are also part of the ACT model... thus, this finding is a confirmation of the model itself in essences). Consider this research, for example: Levitt, J. T., Brown, T. A., Orsillo, S. M. & Barlow, D. H. (2015). (2004). The impact of tolerance and repression of anger on the threat of carbon dioxide in patients with panic disorder, on psychological and psychophysiological reaction. Compliance Treatment, 35, 747-766. In it, acceptance methods (directly drawn from the ACT book) did a better job than control strategies in promoting successful CO_2 gas exposure in patients with panic disorder.

In Campbell-Sills, L., Barlow, D. H., Brown, T. A., & Hofmann, S. G., a comparable finding was accounted for. (2015). (2006). Impacts of concealment and acknowledgment of people with tension and state of mind issue on passionate reactions. Research and Therapy in Behavior, 44, 1251-1263. Similarly, as with the above investigation, brief acknowledgment techniques prompted lower pulse during introduction to an aversive film and more positive impact during the post-film recuperation period that controlled methodologies in on edge and temperament cluttered people.

So far, it looks as if ACT may have a small advantage over traditional CBT methods in outcomes; there is a different set of processes involved in change, and ACT methods may empower traditional behavioral methods.

Theoretically, these are the ACT model's strengths as compared to CBT.

1. The model is scalable and widely applicable. When you look at the entire outcome research that has been published so far (RCTs, regulated time series designs, and case studies), the identified issues shape a fairly broad list: PTSD, hysteria, insomnia, racial bias, burnout, addiction, OCD, stress, paranoia, disease, diabetes, multiple sclerosis, sports psychology, pharmacotherapy behaviors, skin selection, learning new techniques at work, opioid psychology

2. The putative processes of change are well defined in most areas with at least marginally adequate measures available. Such mechanisms of transition are a small set and do not vary wildly from disorder to disorder.

3. This seems the mediational analyzes are effective. Our count has already reported or completed 16 effective systematic mediational analyzes. The results so far are really positive. The mechanisms that have been tested extensively so far include recognition, defusion, beliefs, determined intervention, and psychological resilience so that most of the main ACTs have some evidence in mediational trials.

4. When tested inductively, particular components seem to work. There are at least 18 reports of that type. ACT methods are impactful in every case and work in a theoretically coherent manner. These include all 6 Hexagon concept stages.

5. The basic theory is intricately tied to technology and seems to work itself. For example, we are approaching 10 RFT studies in ACT that are linked to the three senses of self; RFT work is coming on values; and so on.

For those who believe only in manual RCTs, much of that answer will be rejected. But science history shows you can't create a progressive science by using only results studies. In The Scientist-Practitioner I (SCH) explained why (Hayes, Barlow, & Nelson-Gray, 1999). Nevertheless, in a nutshell, it is this: without good theory, the question of technological development is focused on concepts of common sense, and it becomes empirically and theoretically daunting.

This should not be heard as "ACT adherents say RCTs are not important." Nearly 30 RCTs of ACT methods were published by ACT folks. But they don't suffice! Development in the fields of science philosophy, basic principles, applied theory, process specification of change, and efficacy is just as important (and more important in the long term) as technology efficacy tests.

The scientific game played by the ACT / RFT / Contextual Psychology group is this: to try to create a truly progressive psychology science that can more adequately address the human condition. Yes, that's daring, but why don't they have confident objectives? Does the ACT group stand or fall on RCTs as a measure of success? In the end, indeed. But we want and claim yet another, even more challenging criteria: the consequence is to see a more truly useful psychology surface. That includes principles, ideas, materials, basics, efficacy, preparation, distribution, etc.

We believe it is only fair to insist that when considering the progress of this effort, ACT be measured against its own, very difficult criteria. Examining ACT without examining RFT, for example, is like looking at a cancer drug without looking at the physiology.

Like hare and tortoise, ACT follows a slow and steady course. We believe that traditional CBT hopped ahead into a lay cognition theory— which produced rapid progress but long-term problems. We'd rather take the slow path of descriptive behavioral science, one step at a time. Which one goes the farthest? Let's have a feel. Let's be careful and have a peek.

The chances are you've heard in one way or another about cognitive behavioral therapy (CBT). CBT is a present moment, proof-based treatment that has been around since the 1950s (in its most punctual structure) with attention on helping individuals challenge and change ruinous idea examples and conduct.

Acceptance and commitment therapy (ACT— pronounced as the word ' act' rather than the letters) may be less familiar to you—for no other reason than that it has simply not been around for so long. ACT is considered a "third wave" therapy—therapies that go beyond the more traditional cognitive therapies and incorporate other skills into the mix (e.g., awareness, visualization, personal values, etc.) CBT and ACT are both behavior-based therapies but differ primarily from the point of view of thinking. While CBT works by helping you identify and change negative or destructive thoughts, ACT maintains that pain and discomfort are a fact of life—something we need to be comfortable with if we want a happy, fulfilled life to live. That's why ACT encourages you to accept all thoughts instead of trying to change them—both the good and the bad.

We're going to dig a little deeper into both approaches and what sets them apart to get a better understanding of how this looks in therapy.

What is the basic meaning of ACT therapy?

"The only way out is through"—Robert Frost
Consider if she would just like to accept life as it is—the good and the bad—instead of resisting it? That's exactly the point of this type of therapy.

At its core, ACT is a mindfulness-based therapy with the primary objective of enhancing psychological flexibility and helping you build a life that fits your values and authentically feels you.

Using acceptance, commitment, awareness skills, and behavior-changing strategies, ACT's focus is on helping you accept life's realities and accepting thoughts for what they are—just thoughts.

This type of therapy is especially helpful if you are inclined to shy away from the problems of life or avoid them. That is on the grounds that it urges you to draw in with your issues head-on and draw nearer to troublesome emotions, instead of attempting to get them away from them.

How does that look in practice?

ACT teaches you how to make your thoughts more inquisitive, as well as techniques for how to diffuse them.

Different techniques for this could include: repeatedly saying a difficult thought until its meaning disappears and only the sound remains.
To strive to accept a feeling for what it is. For starters, shifting "No one likes me" to "I'm feeling..." teaches you how to develop a relationship with the issues you're dealing with, rather than battling against, such as depression.
The commitment to take action and bring positive changes to your life is another important aspect of ACT. ACT therapy will help you understand the things that matter to you and create a plan that matches your values—and ultimately brings more meaning and purpose into your life.

CBTTherapy; what does it mean?

"Men are disturbed not by things, but by the view they take of them" –Epictetus CBT is a short-term therapy (ACT can be delivered both in the short and long term) that centers on the idea that it is not the events of life itself that cause us problems, but rather the way we interpret them. In other words, the way we think of the world affects our behavior-and ultimately how we feel.

One example could be: if you always anticipate the worst (instead of focusing on the positive), then you will end up being very cautious in life. This kind of thinking is limiting because you are likely to be held back from achieving your goals. This, in turn, will likely leave you feeling sad and unfulfilled.

Thoughts that seem to begin as innocent can easily get ingrained, distorting our world view.

CBT aims to identify and replace those distortions with more positive and rational ways of thinking. And when thoughts change, usually behavior and feelings follow suit.

Because of the nature of this therapy style, it is expected that you will play an active role throughout your sessions, such as homework, learning, and skills training, etc. This could also include tracking mood changes as a way to help you identify problematic patterns of thought and behavior.

Goal-oriented in its approach, you'll leave your initial assessment with a set plan and a clear understanding of how many sessions it will take you to reach your goals (anywhere between 6–20 sessions).

Both ACT and CBT, more or less, are amazing, proof-based treatments that can achieve significant life changes. At last, it's everything about finding a methodology that resounds most with you.

Conclusion

The central origination of Acceptance and Commitment Therapy (ACT) is that mental enduring is generally brought about by the interface between human language and discernment, and the control of human conduct by direct understanding. Mental firmness is contended to rise up out of experiential shirking, subjective trap, connection of a conceptualized self, loss of contact with the present, and the subsequent inability to make required conduct strides as per guiding principle. Buttressed by a broad essential research program on a related hypothesis of language and cognizance, Relational Frame Theory (RFT), ACT takes the view that attempting to change troublesome considerations and sentiments as a methods for adapting can be counter gainful, however new, amazing choices are including acceptance, mindfulness, cognitive defusion, values, and committed action all of which are discussed in this book.